Emergency Action Plan
CPR

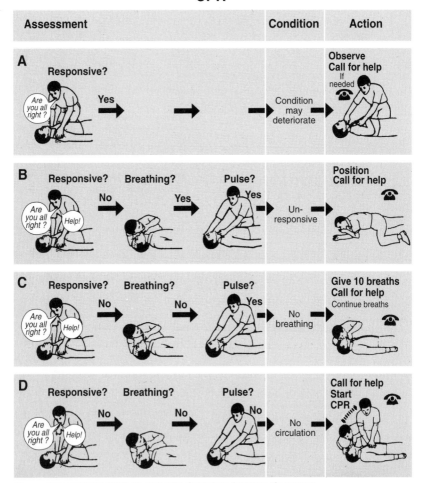

Source: Resuscitation 1992, 24,103–110. Guidelines for basic life support.

OXFORD HANDBOOKS IN EMERGENCY MEDICINE
Series Editors R. N. Illingworth, C. E. Robertson, and M. Clancy

OXFORD HANDBOOKS IN EMERGENCY MEDICINE

This series has already established itself as the essential reference series for staff in A & E departments.

Each book begins with an introduction to the topic, including epidemiology where appropriate. The clinical presentation and the immediate practical management of common conditions are described in detail, enabling the casualty officer or nurse to deal with the problem on the spot. Where appropriate a specific course of action is recommended for each situation and alternatives discussed. Information is clearly laid out and easy to find—important for situations where swift action may be vital.

Details on when, how, and to whom to refer patients are covered, as well as the information required at referral, and what this information is used for. The management of the patient after referral to a specialist is also outlined.

The text of each book is supplemented with checklists, key points, clear diagrams illustrating practical procedures, and recommendations for further reading.

The Oxford Handbooks in Emergency Medicine are an invaluable resource for every member of the A & E team, written and edited by clinicians at the sharp end.

Cardiopulmonary Resuscitation

Second Edition

David V. Skinner

Consultant, Accident and Emergency Medicine,
Clinical Director,
Accident and Emergency Unit,
John Radcliffe Hospital,
Oxford

and

Richard Vincent

Director, Trafford Centre for Medical Research,
University of Sussex;
Consultant Cardiologist, Royal Sussex
County Hospital, Brighton

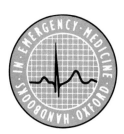

Oxford • New York • Melbourne
OXFORD UNIVERSITY PRESS
1997

Oxford University Press, Walton Street, Oxford OX2 6DP
Oxford   New York
Athens   Auckland   Bangkok   Bombay
Calcutta   Cape Town   Dar es Salaam   Delhi
Florence   Hong Kong   Istanbul   Karachi
Kuala Lumpur   Madras   Madrid   Melbourne
Mexico City   Nairobi   Paris   Singapore
Taipei   Tokyo   Toronto
and associated companies in
Berlin   Ibadan

Oxford is a trade mark of Oxford University Press

Published in the United States
by Oxford University Press Inc., New York

First edition 1993
Second edition 1997

A catalogue record for this book is available from the British Library

Library of Congress Cataloging in Publication Data
Skinner, David V.
Cardiopulmonary resuscitation / David V. Skinner and Richard
Vincent. 2nd ed.
(Oxford handbooks in emergency medicine; 16)
Includes bibliographical references and index.
1. Cardiovascular emergencies.   2. CPR (First aid)   I. Vincent,
Richard (Richard I.)   II. Title.   III. Series.
[DNLM: 1. Cardiopulmonary Resuscitation.   2. Heart arrest–
–therapy.   WB 39 098 v. 16 1996]
RC675.S54   1996   616.1'025–dc20
ISBN 0 19 262694 9 (h/bk).
ISBN 0 19 262693 0 (p/bk).

Typeset by Footnote Graphics, Warminster, Wilts
Printed in Great Britain by
Biddles Ltd
Guildford & King's Lynn

Preface

The management of a patient suffering sudden cardiorespiratory arrest presents a major challenge. In the ensuing few minutes numerous theoretical and practical skills must be brought to bear by a well-ordered team of doctors and nurses in order to give the patient the best chance of survival. The potential for chaos is enormous. The reward for good performance by the team is patient survival and the satisfaction of a job well done.

In 1987 the Royal College of Physicians made detailed recommendations regarding the training of medical students and hospital doctors including, amongst others, the appointment of District Resuscitation Training Officers. This report followed the publication of several studies showing poor performance by junior hospital doctors in resuscitation skills. Rightly, it was perceived that the results of such studies were due to inadequate training.

The European Resuscitation Council has published detailed guidelines for the management of cardiac arrest and, in particular, the treatment of ventricular fibrillation, asystole, and electromechanical dissociation. More recently, the ERC has provided recommendations for the treatment of a broader range of arrhythmias associated with cardiac arrest. It is, therefore, possible to offer didactic guidelines for the management of these emergencies, based on as much scientific data as is currently available.

This book provides all the theoretical knowledge required to manage a cardiorespiratory arrest successfully, as well as other life-threatening cardiac events. It details the organization necessary throughout a hospital district, as well as in different specific areas. A chapter on paediatric resuscitation is included.

It is only through such theoretical learning, reinforced by the assimilation of practical skills, that doctors and nurses can feel sure that every effort has been expended in attempting to resuscitate the unfortunate victim of a cardiorespiratory arrest.

Oxford   D.V.S.
Brighton   R.V.
June 1996

Acknowledgements

Figures 2.1, 2.3, 2.5, 2.7, 6.1, 6.2, 6.3
Reproduced from Evans (1986) with kind permission of the *British Medical Journal*

Figure 3.1
Adapted from Senior (1988).

Figure 5.7
Reproduced from the ISIS-2 Collaborative Group (1988) with permission.

Figure 6.6, 6.8, 6.9, 6.10, 6.11
Reproduced from Skinner *et al.* (1991) with permission.

Figure 7.13
Trace reproduced with kind permission of Dr D. A. Chamberlain.

Figure 7.19
Reproduced with permission of S&R Vickers Ltd.

Figure 8.1
Reproduced with permission from Saunders *et al.* (1988).

Figure 8.2
Reproduced with permission from Brown and Norman (1990).

Figure 8.5
Reproduced from Stanton *et al.* (1989) with permission from the American College of Cardiology (*Journal of the American College of Cardiology*, **14**, 209–15).

Figure 9.8
Reproduced from Oakley (1988) with kind permission of the *British Medical Journal*.

Box 8.4 Data from Weil *et al.* (1985)

Front endpaper
Reproduced from *Resuscitation* (1992), **24**, 103–10, with permission.

Back endpaper
Reproduced with kind permission of Resuscitation Council (UK).

Contents

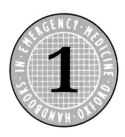

Introduction to cardiopulmonary resuscitation

Key points in an introduction to cardiopulmonary resuscitation

1 Fifty per cent of those who die of myocardial infarction do so within 2 hours of the onset of symptoms.

2 Many patients in the community experiencing sudden cardiac death have few or no warning symptoms.

3 Public awareness of the signs and symptoms of acute myocardial infarction remain poor.

4 Early deaths during myocardial infarction are usually due to ventricular fibrillation.

5 Recent educational initiatives should improve the previously low standard of resuscitation skills among hospital doctors.

Epidemiology

In the United Kingdom approximately 160 000 deaths occur each year as a result of coronary artery disease; in the United States the annual mortality from this condition is around 650 000. Although trauma is the commonest cause of death in the first four decades of life, coronary artery disease rapidly overtakes trauma as a killer and, in later years, competes with malignancy as the leading cause of death.

The incidence of coronary artery disease in the United Kingdom varies geographically, being about twice as common in the west of Scotland as in the south-east of England. Recognized risk factors include increasing age, smoking, hypertension, high serum lipid levels, diabetes, and familial factors. Men are affected four times more frequently than women, and recent evidence suggests that coronary disease is more common among social classes IV and V than in social classes I and II.

Coronary artery disease is responsible for acute myocardial infarction and for sudden cardiac death without muscle damage. Between 40 and 50 per cent of those suffering myocardial infarction die within 20 days of the attack. Of 100 patients suffering an acute myocardial infarction 75 reach hospital alive, and only 62 leave hospital. Seven of these survivors are destined to die in the first year after discharge. Fifty per cent of those who die, do so within the first two hours after the onset of symptoms, and many suffering sudden death have no warning symptoms at all. Up to 70 per cent fail to reach hospital. The management of such early deaths following the onset of symptoms remains a challenge for all involved in the care of patients with acute coronary syndromes. Early recognition of such ischaemic episodes by the patient, bystanders, the general practitioners and hospital doctors is the key to improving survival rates.

Chain of survival

It is now generally agreed, particularly with the advent of thrombolytic therapy, that patients with acute myocardial infarction are best managed in hospital-based cardiac care units. However, to address the threat of early fatal arrhythmias there must also be provision of skilled help in the community—from general practitioners, from local resuscitation ambulances, or from ordinary ambulances equipped with automated defibrillators and other resuscitation equipment, with crews experienced in their use. Of further value is a general awareness in the population of the hazards of acute myocardial infarction, together with a knowledge of the symptoms of a typical attack. Such educational initiatives should ideally take place in school. Public education is essential if myocardial infarction is to be recognized early. Cardiopulmonary resuscitation (CPR) can also be commenced by a bystander if collapse occurs before the arrival of the ambulance. The prompt arrival of defibrillator-trained ambulance personnel is vital if survival is to be maximized. Calling for help is the first element of the 'chain of survival' (Box 1.1)—a sequence of events which is the key to the successful recovery from rescuable causes of circulatory arrest.

Box 1.1 ● The Chain of Survival

Early access
Early BLS
Early defibrillation
Early ALS

BLS, basic life support.
ALS, advanced (cardiac) life support.

The cause of death in patients suffering cardiac arrest following the onset of acute myocardial infarction or ischaemia is usually a malignant ventricular arrhythmia—most commonly ventricular fibrillation. This fact is particularly distressing in that with early defibrillation many of these patients can be saved. A patient developing ventricular fibrillation will rapidly start to feel faint and lose consciousness, collapsing to the floor. Effective cardiac output ceases, and, within half a minute, normal respiration ceases, although intermittent 'gasping' respiratory movements can persist for several minutes following cardiac arrest. Unless prompt and effective resuscitation and defibrillation are readily to hand, the patient will die.

Public education and pre-hospital care

Maximizing survival from the devastating effects of coronary disease depends on increasing awareness among the general public of the presentation of myocardial infarction and of the need for urgent admission to hospital—usually via the ambulance system alone, but, in some areas, in association with a rapidly responding, defibrillator-carrying general practitioner.

The public must also know the practical measures to take if an individual collapses before the arrival of the emergency services. Eisenberg showed that the timely intervention of a bystander and the rapid availability of a defibrillator gave the best results for those suffering from ventricular fibrillation. Provision of basic life support (chest compression and ventilation) within four minutes of collapse, and delivery of advanced life support (notably defibrillation) within eight minutes resulted in the survival to hospital discharge of around 45 per cent of patients presenting in ventricular fibrillation.

The need to provide skilled resuscitation facilities before arrival at hospital was addressed nearly thirty years ago. The first mobile coronary care unit was launched by Pantridge and Geddes in Belfast in 1966. The ambulance carried a doctor and nurse together with a portable defibrillator, and successfully resuscitated patients who clearly would otherwise have died. A combined approach by Chamberlain and his colleagues has been to train ambulance personnel to a high level of expertise in cardiopulmonary resuscitation, defibrillation, and drug administration, together with a large community resuscitation training programme which continues to alert the general public to the actions to be taken in the presence of myocardial infarction and cardiac arrest. The training of ambulance personnel nationally to paramedic standard has now been adopted by the National Health Service Training Directorate.

Pai studied the effectiveness in a rural community of GPs equipped with defibrillators in dealing with 1011 heart attacks. The 28-day mortality was 36 per cent, and 59 per cent of deaths occurred outside hospital. The GP was the first medical contact in 92 per cent of heart attacks, and was equipped with a defibrillator in 80 per cent of such cases. Of those who had a cardiac arrest in the presence of a GP equipped with a defibrillator 28 per cent survived until they left hospital (Figure 1.1).

More recently, the optimum medical treatment of cardiopulmonary arrest from any cause has received detailed attention from specialist groups in the United Kingdom and abroad. Protocols for basic and advanced life support have been agreed internationally, and are now readily available to the medical and lay communities. Major problems remain in the education and logistics needed to deliver effective resuscitation throughout the United Kingdom. In spite of focused attempts at community education, the skill and enthusiasm

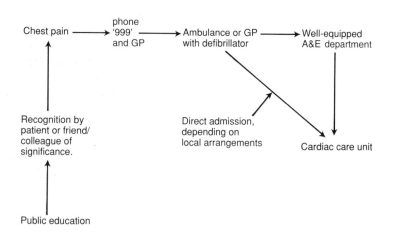

Thrombolysis, where appropriate, depending on local arrangements at any stage from '999' onwards.

Fig. 1.1 ● Flowchart for the ideal management of a patient with chest pain.

of the general public in the recognition of acute coronary syndromes and the delivery of adequate basic life support is patchy.

Resuscitation training in hospital

The resuscitation skills of hospital doctors, general practitioners, and nursing staff of all grades are often poor. It has been shown that there is an appalling lack of skills in both basic life support (BLS) and advanced (cardiac) life support (ALS) among hospital doctors and nurses. Either a partial or a complete lack of practical knowledge of external cardiac massage and mouth-to-mouth breathing is common among doctors. Intubation skills have been shown to be universally poor. This reflected a general paucity in training within the medical school curriculum. However, this situation should improve with the increasing availability of ALS training.

In addition the Royal Colleges, the British Heart Foundation, the ambulance authorities, and the Resuscitation Council (UK) have recognized the need for increased training of professionals in resuscitation techniques, and have been responsible for new educational initiatives. Increasing emphasis is also being placed on the organizational requirements for rapid delivery of cardiopulmonary support, both in the community and in hospital. These new attitudes in education and organization will bring a marked increase in the number of lives saved. The work of Eisenberg and colleagues has shown that the intervention of a trained bystander could potentially double the survival from out-of-hospital cardiac arrest due to ventricular fibrillation.

Further reading

1. Casey, W. F. (1984). Cardiopulmonary resuscitation: a survey of standards among junior hospital doctors. *Journal of the Royal Society of Medicine*, **77**, 921–4.
2. Cummins, R. O., Ornato, J. P., Thies, W. K., and Pepe, P. E. (1991). Improving the survival from sudden cardiac arrest: the 'chain of survival' concept. *Circulation*, **83**, 1832–47.

3. Eisenberg, M. S., Bergner, L., and Hallstrom, A. P. (1979). Cardiac resuscitation in the community. *Journal of the American Medical Association*, **241**, 1905–7.
4. Hearne, T. R. and Cummins, R. O. (1988). Improved survival from cardiac arrest in the community. *Pacing and Clinical Electrophysiology*, **11**, 1968–73.
5. Pai, G. R., Haites, N. E., and Rawles, J. M. (1987). 1000 heart attacks in Grampian: the place of CPR in general practice. *British Medical Journal*, **294**, 352–4.
6. Pantridge, J. F. and Geddes, J. S. (1967). A mobile intensive care unit in the management of myocardial infarction. *Lancet*, **ii**, 271–3.
7. Royal College of Physicians (1987). Resuscitation from cardiopulmonary arrest. Training and organisation. *Journal of the Royal College of Physicians, London*, **21**, 1–8.
8. Seidelin, P. H., McMurray, J. J. V., Stolarek, I. H., and Robertson, C. E. (1989). The basic and advanced cardiopulmonary resuscitation skills of trained nursing staff. *Scottish Medical Journal*, **34**, 393–4.
9. Skinner, D. V., Camm, A. J., and Miles, S. (1985). Cardiopulmonary resuscitation skills of pre-registration house officers. British Medical Journal, **290**, 1549–50.
10. Vincent, R., Martin, B., Williams, G., Quinn, E., Robertson, G., and Chamberlain, D. A. (1984). A community training scheme in cardiopulmonary resuscitation. *British Medical Journal*, **288**, 617–20.
11. Weston, C. F. M., Penny, W. J., and Julian, D. G. (1994). Guidelines for the early management of patients with myocardial infarction. *British Medical Journal*, **308**, 767–71.

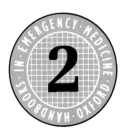

CHAPTER 2

Management of cardiac arrest

Key points in the management of cardiac arrest

1 Cardiopulmonary resuscitation should be conducted in a calm, quiet, structured fashion.

2 The 'team leader' should be minimally involved in practical procedures.

3 Ventricular fibrillation is more amenable to treatment than asystole or electromechanical dissociation.

4 In ventricular fibrillation, the earlier the defibrillating shock is given, the better the result. The effectiveness of defibrillation falls rapidly with even small delays to treatment.

5 Apparent asystole may be fine ventricular fibrillation—look carefully.

6 Electromechanical dissociation may be primary, and rarely treatable, or secondary, and potentially treatable.

7 A prolonged resuscitation attempt is rarely associated with survival to leave hospital.

8 Open cardiac massage is more effective, but much less practicable, than external cardiac massage—there are, however, specific indications.

Recognition of cardiac arrest

The diagnosis of cardiac arrest is a clinical one, and is confirmed if the patient is both unconscious and pulseless. The absence of a major (i.e. carotid or femoral) pulse in a patient who fails to respond to gentle shaking and a loud voice is the key finding.

Other clinical 'features' of cardiac arrest are unreliable, and to look for them wastes precious time. Thus, ineffectual gasping respirations may persist for several minutes after cardiac arrest, and pupil size and the presence of cyanosis or pallor are also unreliable and unnecessary as a guide to the diagnosis of an arrest (although a note at the outset may be helpful for later comparison).

A patient in cardiac arrest may occasionally present as a *grand mal* convulsion. Initially, this may be misleading. Tonic contractions may be marked; but clonic movements are minor or absent, and the patient will be profoundly cyanosed. The fit will be short-lived. Wait for it to subside (protecting the patient from injury if necessary), and then check for a major pulse.

The diagnosis of cardiac arrest in a patient attached to an electrocardiograph (ECG) monitor is usually straightforward, but beware a broken connection giving erroneous 'asystole', or skeletal muscle potentials mimicking ventricular fibrillation.

Treat the patient, not the electrocardiograph

Once the diagnosis of cardiac arrest is made, a decision must be taken rapidly as to whether or not to commence resuscitation.

Should resuscitation proceed?

For in-patients a decision should have been made beforehand, by the consultant in charge of the case, his team, relatives, and, if appropriate, the patient about whether or not to resuscitate; cardiac arrest teams should not have to make decisions in seconds, with little or no knowledge of patients and their illnesses. Four potential reasons for limiting treatment which have been suggested are: that the patient declines; that the treatment is futile; that the costs are too great; or that the quality of life would be unacceptable.

For patients brought to an accident and emergency department with cardiac arrest or whose arrest occurs within minutes of arrival, resuscitation must always be commenced, as basic facts, such as the cause of the arrest, the patient's age, the previous duration of the arrest, or the immediate medical history, are often unavailable. A rapid history should be sought from the ambulance crew and any accompanying relatives or friends. Clearly, resuscitation must not be delayed; but enthusiasm for a prolonged attempt should be tempered in the light of adverse features in the history (see p. 25).

Box 2.1 • Information required from relatives/ambulance staff

- Time of collapse
- Age
- Past medical history
- Current medication
- Chest pain before arrest/collapse
- Bystander CPR
- Ambulance CPR
- Ambulance ALS

Management of cardiac arrest in hospital

The sequence of events when dealing with a cardiac arrest occurring in hospital is as follows:

First, call for help/arrest team and commence basic life support (BLS), ideally with a Laerdal pocket mask for ventilation and external chest compression.

Then, if the cause or duration of the arrest is uncertain, the conventional order of **A**irway, **B**reathing, and **C**irculation is appropriate.

For a patient whose collapse is witnessed and therefore likely to be due to ventricular fibrillation, give a precordial thump, check the pulse again, and, if it is absent, begin basic life support with 15–30 chest compressions before the need for ventilation; the order is then; **C, A, B**. The rationale of this recommendation is that at the moment of collapse in a patient with unheralded ventricular fibrillation, the lungs and the arterial blood are well oxygenated. Primary circulatory arrest has occurred, for which the most urgent treatment is restoration of the circulation—by chest compression and urgent defibrillation.

This sequence differs from the universal protocol suggested by the European Resuscitation Council (UK), but is offered as a logical alternative for those providing *skilled* aid.

Basic life-support techniques

Box 2.2 ● Calling the crash team

1. Ring XXXX
2. 'Cardiac arrest on Nightingale Ward'

---

1. Begin basic life support and call for the 'crash' team. The technique of basic life support is straightforward; but some practical points are worth emphasis. Opening the airway is best achieved by head tilt and chin lift or jaw thrust techniques. A Laerdal pocket mask (Fig. 6.4, p. 102) with expired air respiration is easier to use than the more familiar bag-and-mask technique, especially for one-person resuscitation.

    Chest compression must be given using a vertical force in the midline. Deliver downward pressure with a rhythmic rather than jerky action, using straight arms and the heel of the hand on the lower half of the patient's sternum, and depressing to a depth of one and a half to two inches. The fingers should be kept well away from the chest wall. (Fig. 2.1)

2. Give 15 compressions to 2 inflations for a single attendant, or 5 compressions to 1 inflation where two helpers are present. When there are two attendants performing resuscitation the person providing external cardiac compression should pause after each 5th compression to allow adequate lung inflation by the other attendant.

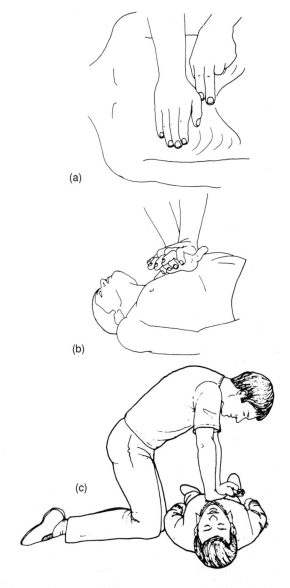

(a)

(b)

(c)

Fig. 2.1 • (a) finding the correct hand position for external chest compression (ECC). (b) Two interlocked hands in position ready to commence ECC. (c) Position of patient and rescuer during ECC.

3. Send staff to collect: 1. CRASH BOX (Table 2.1)
                                 2. DEFIBRILLATOR

4. On arrival of the crash team:

Table 2.1 ● Suggested contents for a hospital crash box

---

1 × size 7.0 ET Tube
1 × size 8.0 ET Tube
1 × size 9.0 ET Tube
(NB: All tubes pre-cut to length)
1 endotracheal adaptor set
Gum elastic bougie
Magill forceps
Macintosh laryngoscope + spare bulb/batteries
1 × 10 ml syringe
Size 2, 3, and 4 Guedel airways
Laerdal pocket mask (should be available before the
  crash team arrives)
1 giving set
500 ml dextrose 5%

1 emergency drug box containing:

1 × adrenaline 1:1000	10 mg/10 ml
4 × adrenaline 1:10000	1mg/10 ml
3 × atropine sulphate	1mg/10 ml
2 × calcium chloride 10%	10 ml
2 × lignocaine hydrochloride 1%	100 mg/10 ml
1 × sodium bicarbonate 8.4%	50 ml

2 × 3-way tap with extensiion
Cannulae
2 × size 14G (5¼″ long)
2 × size 16G (standard)
2 × size 18G (standard)
2 × size 20G (standard)
1 size 12/14G cannula over needle for crithyroidotomy
2 sterile gauze packs
2 dressings
1 roll adhesive tape—1 inch (25 mm) wide
1 self-inflating bag + size 4 and 5 facemasks
1 bandage
1 Yankauer sucker
Oxygen tubing
Soft/flexible suction catheters
–2 × 12 gauge
–2 × 14 gauge

Advanced cardiac life support

The team should be organized rapidly by the team leader (TL). The specialty of the TL is not important, and he or she may be from anaesthetics, general medicine, accident and emergency, or cardiology. Most importantly, however, the TL should only be minimally involved in the practicalities of treatment. The TL must have sufficient experience and sensitivity to direct the other team members in a structured and predetermined pattern. The TL should usually be of Registrar/Senior Registrar grade.

Box 2.3 ● Role of the team leader

During the arrest
● Assume control and organize the team
● Co-ordinate everyone's efforts
● Receive input from team members and make decisions regarding treatment, including, if necessary, termination of the arrest attempt

After the attempt
● Ensure proper handover to in-patient team if the patient survives
● Discuss the result of the resuscitation attempt with the relatives
● Organize a 'review' of the team's efforts

Cardiac arrest team organization

Shown in Fig. 2.2 are the suggested roles of the various team members.

As soon as the monitor is attached the underlying arrest rhythm should be assessed by the TL—external cardiac compression should cease for a moment, but for no longer than 10 seconds at a time. Treatment should then continue depending on the rhythm, according to the guidelines of the European Resuscitation Council; the three main rhythms likely to be encountered are:

1. ventricular fibrillation/pulseless ventricular tachycardia (VT);

2. (EMD) (primary or secondary); and
3. asystole.

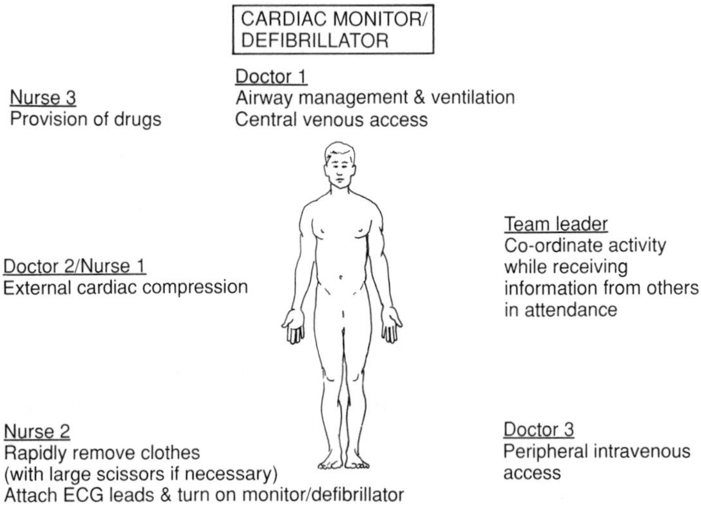

CARDIAC MONITOR/
DEFIBRILLATOR

Nurse 3
Provision of drugs

Doctor 1
Airway management & ventilation
Central venous access

Team leader
Co-ordinate activity
while receiving
information from others
in attendance

Doctor 2/Nurse 1
External cardiac compression

Nurse 2
Rapidly remove clothes
(with large scissors if necessary)
Attach ECG leads & turn on monitor/defibrillator

Doctor 3
Peripheral intravenous
access

Fig. 2.2 ● Suggested roles of the team leader (TL) and team members.

Box 2.4 ● General rules for team/team leader

● Whole arrest should be conducted in calm, quiet, confident manner
● No 'breakaway' diagnosis or treatment groups
● Interruptions of chest compression should always be *limited*
● Consider team safety
– gloves/aprons/glasses
– defibrillator (inadvertent contact, defibrillator not discharged after shock deemed unnecessary)
– blood/fluid on floor

Box 2.5 • Tasks commenced simultaneously on diagnosis of cardiac arrest by crash team

- Secure airway and commence ventilation
- Commence external chest compression
- Clothes off—monitor/defibrillator leads on
- Defibrillation as soon as VF/pulseless VT is confirmed
- Insert peripheral/central intravenous lines

Management of life-threatening arrhythmias

Ventricular fibrillation (VF)

This is most easily corrected when a DC shock is delivered with minimal delay (Figs 2.3 and 2.4). Hence the immediate availability of a defibrillator, and its early use, is vital. The paddles of the defibrillator should be placed on the patient with the object of enclosing as much ventricular muscle as possible between them. The standard positions are the right subclavicular area, and just outside the cardiac apex (V4–5), as shown in Fig. 2.5. Gel pads must be placed in position before the defibrillator paddles are applied to the chest wall. Front-to-back is a more effective position electrically, but is impractical for the supine patient. Paddle placement should

---

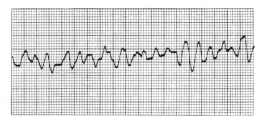

Fig. 2.3 • Ventricular fibrillation.

avoid monitoring electrodes, breast tissue, GTN patches (which may explode!), and permanent pacemaker generators. (If the presenting rhythm is VF, an external DC shock is required even in the presence of a permanent pacing system or an internal defibrillator.)

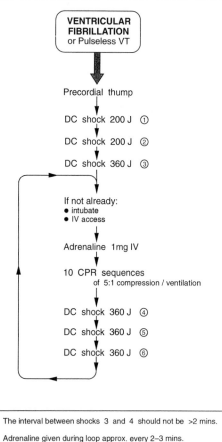

Fig. 2.4 • Flowchart for the management of ventricular fibrillation/pulseless ventricular tachycardia.

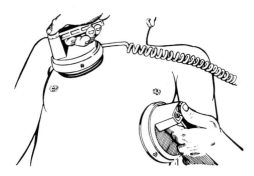

Fig. 2.5 ● Defibrillator paddle position during defibrillation.

Good contact with the chest should be ensured by allowing the paddles to be on as flat an area of the chest as possible, the use of pre-gelled pads (safer than jelly), and firm perpendicular pressure on each electrode. Avoid undue tension in the wires.

Defibrillation The first three shocks are given as quickly as possible with a pause between them sufficient only to:

(a) check the pulse
(b) confirm that the rhythm is still VF/VT, and the patient is still pulseless
(c) recharge defibrillator.

Basic life support should be given between shocks only if the charge time is slow (>15 sec) and should never delay the application of the next shock in the sequence.

Following effective cardioversion there is an electrical delay in restoring a recordable rhythm, and there can be a mechanical delay in the restoration of effective cardiac output.

The recommended energy for the first two shocks is the same (200 J); but their effects may differ. If unsuccessful in defibrillating, the first shock will reduce tissue impedance and allow a greater current flow during the second shock. The effect of the second shock may also be cumulative with that of the first in reducing the amount of myocardium involved in the arrhythmia mechanism until it is below the 'critical mass' necessary to sustain ventricular fibrillation.

Drug administration in ventricular fibrillation If three promptly administered DC shocks fail to restore a co-ordinated rhythm, then the arrest is likely to be prolonged. At this stage—if this has not been done already—the patient should be intubated, positive-pressure ventilation should commence, intravenous (IV) access should be secured, and emergency drugs should be prepared. Basic life support should not be interrupted during these procedures for more than 15 seconds. The first drug of choice is **adrenaline 1 mg** (10 ml of a 1:10 000 solution), given centrally if possible. Its use is to increase the efficiency of basic life support in achieving coronary and cerebral perfusion, rather than as a specific aid to defibrillation. Ten sequences of five compressions to one ventilation are now applied before a further set of three DC shocks, all at 360 J. If VF remains refractory the loop (Fig. 2.4) is repeated each time including adrenaline 1 mg. After **every 3 loops** an alkalizing agent (e.g. sodium bicarbonate 50 mEq) is *considered* as is the use of anti-arrhythmic agents, lignocaine, bretylium, or amiodarone.

Management of persistent ventricular fibrillation For VF that persists, the use of an alternative defibrillator, new paddle positions (perhaps front-to-back), or even a double-shock technique is suggested. The use of various anti-arrhythmic drugs in persistent ventricular fibrillation is discussed in Chapter 8.

Electromechanical dissociation (EMD)

EMD is a clinical condition of cardiac arrest with no palpable cardiac output in spite of ordered ventricular electrical activity. This may be 'primary' EMD, a result of the failure of the myocardium to respond to electrical stimulation; or secondary, as the result of conditions such as hypovolaemia, pneumothorax, cardiac tamponade, or pulmonary embolus (Fig. 2.6).

EMD occurs commonly for a short period after defibrillation; and in this situation the remedy is patience with continued basic life support until cardiac output returns.

Other aetiologies, some of which are potentially treatable, include:

• severe hypovolaemia (trauma, concealed haemorrhage);
• pneumothorax (bilateral, tension);

(a)   Causes of electromechanical dissociation

Primary
• Electrical activity present but no corresponding effective pumping action by myocardium. This is usually related to massive muscle damage.

Secondary
• Hypovolaemia: exclude on history and examination (remember to do rectal examination for concealed gastrointestinal haemorrhage).
• Cardiac tamponade: *pericardiocentesis*.
• Tension pneumothorax: clinical examination -if correct, needle/drain

(b)

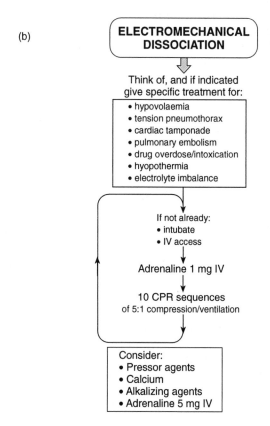

Fig. 2.6 ● (a) Electromechanical dissociation (EMD) classification. (b) Flowchart for the management of EMD.

- cardiac tamponade (infarction with myocardial rupture, trauma);
- massive pulmonary embolism;
- hypothermia; and
- profound electrolyte disturbance.

Consider specific therapies from the outset, especially volume replacement for hypovolaemia, pericardial tap for tamponade, and the urgent treatment of tension pneumothorax. The use of centrally administered thrombolytic agents for massive pulmonary embolism is currently under consideration, but has not become routine practice.

Drug administration in EMD For EMD with no immediately remediable cause the drug of first choice is adrenaline. Its beneficial action is mediated chiefly through its alpha effect on peripheral vasomotor tone, although beta adrenergic stimulation can be helpful for cardiac support on recovery. The dose is 1 mg given as centrally as possible (see Chapter 8). A higher dose, 5 mg, may be considered if the arrest is prolonged.

Calcium ions play a key role in the heart in linking electrical to mechanical activity; but calcium chloride given exogenously may adversely affect the cellular response to reperfusion, and may hinder neurological outcome. Calcium chloride is recommended only for EMD that is due to hyperkalaemia, hypocalcaemia, or an overdose of calcium-channel blocking agents.

Asystole

Asystole is characterized by an absence of ventricular electrical activity on ECG in the presence of clinical cardiac arrest. Always check that the leads are properly connected to the chest and that the lead select button is appropriately positioned. Note that asystole is rarely a 'straight-line' trace.

The outcome of treating asystole is usually disappointing, especially in severe myocardial ischaemia/infarction, or where the heart shows no sign at all of electrical activity ('asystole without P waves'). The presence of P waves, Fig. 2.7, is more encouraging.

Management of asystole It is important to consider whether the presenting rhythm is in fact fine ventricular fibrillation rather than asystole. If ventricular fibrillation is a possibility the appropriate treatment algorithm (see p. 00) should be applied. For true asystole, early intubation and ventilation are mandatory; in a few cases adequate oxygenation and external chest compression alone are enough to restart the heart. Drug therapy comprises, first, adrenaline 1 mg for its alpha and beta effects, and then (once only and very much as second best) atropine 3 mg. (Figure 2.8).

Transthoracic external pacing can be effective in patients whose hearts show residual electrical activity. But apparent arterial pulsation and ECG artefact may both be produced by this technique in the absence of true myocardial stimulation; improving cerebral perfusion is the best evidence for success. Transthoracic pacing may be useful occasionally to 'cover' the delay until a transvenous pacing system can be established. In the absence of electrical activity, further loops of 1 mg adrenaline and continued CPR are recommended.

When to stop resuscitation

The cause of the arrest, the response to treatment, and the age of the patient are all important factors to consider when deciding when to abandon a resuscitation attempt. Bedell found no survivors among 294 hospital patients who had had cardiac arrest if the resuscitation attempt continued for longer than 30 minutes. However, for patients with cardiac arrest associated with drug overdose, drowning, or hypothermia, and in the young, prolonged resuscitation attempts should be undertaken, and are occasionally successful.

The team's responsibilities for medical care do not end with a successful restoration of spontaneous cardiac output. Imme-

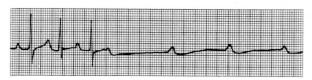

Fig. 2.7 • Onset of ventricular asystole with 'P waves'.

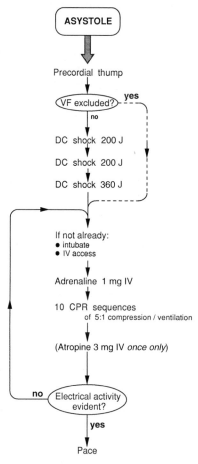

Fig. 2.8 ● Flowchart for the management of asystole.

diate measures include frequent recording of pulse and blood pressure and ECG monitoring. If the patient remains unconscious, airway protection and assisted ventilation will be necessary. Arterial blood gases should be checked, together with urea and electrolytes, particularly serum potassium. The physician responsible for the patient's further care should be clearly identified, and the patient should be promptly transferred to a bed in the intensive care unit.

Internal cardiac massage

Technique

External or closed-chest compression, introduced by Kouwenhoven in 1960, is a convenient technique for maintaining the circulation during ventricular standstill. Cardiac output and cerebral perfusion obtained by this method are, however, poor—usually less than 25 per cent of normal, with carotid flows that may not exceed 10 per cent of basal levels.

True direct cardiac massage using an **open** chest technique has been shown to increase both myocardial and cerebral perfusion in animals and man. It is inevitably more traumatic and less practicable, although the technique is simple.

An incision is made below the left breast in the fourth or fifth intercostal space, one sweep of the scalpel exposing the intercostal muscles. The intercostal muscles are divided by blunt dissection and the ribs are spread (more easily using a mechanical device). The operator's hand is then inserted to cradle the heart in the palm and begin compression against the sternum. The pericardium does not need to be opened unless tamponade is suspected.

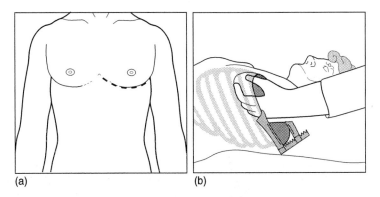

(a) (b)

Fig. 2.9 ● (a) An incision is made below the left breast in the fourth or fifth intercostal space. (b) Open chest cardiac massage.

Indications for the use of internal cardiac massage

The indications for open cardiac massage in non-traumatic cardiac arrest remain controversial. If the technique is to be used, however, it is most effective within 15 minutes of the patient's cardiac arrest (see Safar 1994).

Trauma resuscitation

The resuscitation of a multiply injured patient is complex and challenging. The Royal College of Surgeons' report suggests that 20 per cent of such patients who die do so unnecessarily, because of poor management in hospital. The management of the multiply injured patient is dealt with in a separate book in this OUP series.

Further reading

1. Bedell, S. E., Delbanco, T. L., Cook, E. F., and Epstein, E. F. (1983). Survival after cardiopulmonary resuscitation in hospital. *New England Journal of Medicine*, **309**, 569–76.
2. European Resuscitation Council Basic Life Support Working Group (1993). Guidelines for basic life support. *British Medical Journal*, **300**, 1587–9.
3. Colquhoun, M. C., Handley, A. J., and Evans, T. R. (ed.) (1995). ABC of resuscitation, 3rd edn. British Medical Journal, London.
4. European Resuscitation Council Advanced Life Support Working Group. (1993). Guidelines for Advanced Life Support. *British Medical Journal*, **300**, 1589–93.
5. Kouwenhoven, W. B., Jude, J. R., and Knickerbocker, G. G. (1970). Closed chest cardiac massage. *Journal of the American Medical Association*, **173**, 1064–7.
6. Lo, B. and Jonsen, A. R. (1980). Clinical decisions to limit treatment. *Annals of Internal Medicine*, **99**, 764–8.
7. Robertson, C. and Redmond, A. D. (1994). *The management of major trauma.* Oxford University Press.
8. Royal College of Surgeons (1988). *The management of patients with major injuries.* Report of the Working Party on the Management of Patients with Major Injuries, RCS.
9. Safar, P. (1994). Recent advances in cardiopulmonary cerebral resuscitation. *Annals of Emergency Medicine*, **13**, 856.

10. Weston, C. I. M., Penny, W. J., and Julian, D. G. (1994). Guidelines for the early management of patients with myocardial infarction. *British Medical Journal*, **308**, 767–71.

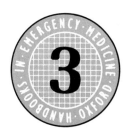

CHAPTER 3

Cardiac arrest associated with special circumstances

Key points in cardiac arrest associated with special circumstances

1 Careful assessment of the immediate history or surroundings is advised to identify any specific cause for a patient's collapse.

2 Airway protection, ventilation, and circulatory support remain central to treatment but with variable emphasis and the inclusion of other treatment modalities according to the special circumstances of the arrest.

3 Support of ventilatory function and adequate oxygenation is the primary need in respiratory arrest, severe bronchospasm, pulmonary embolism, certain causes of drug overdose, and drowning.

4 Correction of hypoxia alone may reverse the progression of a profound bradycardia to asytole.

5 Adrenaline plays a key role in severe resistant bronchospasm in anaphylaxis and major pulmonary embolism.

6 Specific antidotes to ingested poisons are uncommon. Consult a local poison centre for best advice.

7 In late pregnancy resuscitation may be helped by lateral rotation by 30°. Emergency Caesarean section is recommended if resuscitation has been unsuccessful within 5 minutes of collapse.

Introduction

A number of conditions other than major cardiac arrhythmias present with life-threatening disorders of circulatory or respiratory function. They can often be suspected from the patient's immediate history or surroundings, but occasionally the underlying pathology is obscure. Airway protection, ventilation, and circulatory support, as previously described, remain central to their treatment; but particular aspects of diagnosis and management are worth noting.

Primary respiratory arrest

In adults, primary respiratory arrest is uncommon, and usually occurs as a result of intracerebral pathology (e.g. intracranial haemorrhage or raised intracranial pressure), the effect of depressant drugs (e.g. opioids or tricyclic antidepressants), or profound metabolic derangement. Initially, cardiac output will be maintained, but in the face of progressive anoxia heart rate and then myocardial contractility will diminish.

The diagnosis usually rests on the observation of an apnoeic and cyanosed patient, initially with a palpable pulse. In the absence of effective therapy, circulatory failure will follow, associated with vasodilation and profound bradycardia, asystole, or electromechanical dissociation.

The essential requirement is for intubation, oxygenation, and assisted ventilation with chest compression and adrenaline for the patient who is pulseless. If the case is treated promptly, restoration of a satisfactory circulation may follow the introduction of full ventilatory support alone.

Asthma and severe bronchospasm

Asthmatic patients are vulnerable to episodes of severe bronchial narrowing from a combination of spasm and mucous plugging. Several factors may contribute to a rapid deterioration resulting in collapse (Box 3.1). Most commonly, profound hypoxia, the development of respiratory acidosis, and exhaustion lead to marked bradycardia followed by asystole. Ventricular fibrillation may supervene.

Box 3.1 • Contributing factors to circulatory arrest in asthma

- Profound hypoxia
- Respiratory acidosis
- Exhaustion
- Adrenal failure
- Dehydration
- Pneumothorax
- Pneumomediastinum

Support of ventilatory function is the first requirement, with urgent attention to tension pneumothorax if present. (Note that tension pneumothorax is extremely unusual in non-ventilated patients.) Intubate, with suction if necessary; ventilate with 100 per cent oxygen; and confirm the presence of bilateral air entry by observation of chest movement and by auscultation.

Cardiac arrhythmias may be refractory to conventional therapy, and anti-arrhythmic drugs are contraindicated until hypoxia and acid—base status have been restored. In some patients, failure of an endogenous sympatho-adrenal response with an unexpectedly low plasma adrenaline may add to circulatory distress. For these, the early administration of adrenaline is especially helpful. In the face of dehydration the patient may also need fluid replacement to restore plasma volume. In the younger patient, internal cardiac massage should be considered for cardiac arrest resulting from severe asthma. Chest compression may be impeded by the hyperinflated, mucous-plugged lungs, and further increasing intrathoracic pressure by external cardiac compression increases the risk of pneumothorax. Internal cardiac massage provides an effective circulation, while the primary abnormality of gas exchange is slowly corrected.

Pulmonary embolism

Life-threatening pulmonary embolism characteristically causes circulatory arrest with a markedly elevated jugular venous pressure (JVP), deep cyanosis, and an initial tachypnoea before spontaneous respirations fade. At first, a near-normal cardiac rhythm is seen, simulating electromechanical dissociation. But as hypoxia advances the heart slows, often as a prelude to ventricular fibrillation. The appearances are virtually identical to those of pericardial tamponade from ventricular rupture after acute myocardial infarction, and differentiation may be impossible unless the preceding history is clear.

Full cardiopulmonary support will be necessary at once—to deliver high levels of inspired oxygen and to promote a circulation through the pulmonary arterial tree. Adrenaline should be used early to counter bradycardia, enhance right ventricular contraction, and maintain venous tone.

When pulmonary obstruction is severe, cardiac compression is ineffective, and the patient remains suffused, pulseless, and deeply cyanosed. If resuscitation is clearly failing to restore any cardiac output, the attempt need not be unduly prolonged. No other intervention will be helpful at this stage.

If circulatory rescue is possible it will usually be achieved within a few minutes. The major pulmonary clot disperses into distal vessels, and as oxygenation improves pulmonary arteriolar resistance falls.

The treatment of the patient resuscitated from massive pulmonary embolism requires careful consideration. A suggested approach is shown in Fig. 3.1. Where the patient is haemodynamically unstable and has no relevant contraindications, thrombolytic therapy with streptokinase is the treatment of choice. The dose is 250 000 units in the first hour followed by an intravenous infusion of 1 000 000 units per hour for the next 24 hours. (The use of low-dose streptokinase or other thrombolytic agents is currently under review.)

Emergency surgical embolectomy is more difficult to undertake, and is usually preceded by pulmonary angiography to confirm the diagnosis. Mortality is 40 to 50 per cent; and this procedure appears to offer no therapeutic advantage over

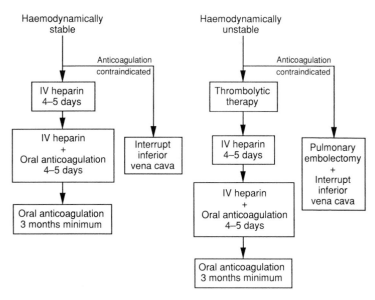

Fig. 3.1 ● Therapy for pulmonary embolism.

thrombolysis. The same can be said of removal of the emboli by a special suction catheter.

Anaphylaxis

Anaphylaxis is an immediate hypersensitivity reaction that can be triggered by a variety of agents (Box 3.2). Within a minute or two of exposure to the offending agent the patient develops the effects of a massive release of histamine from mast cells (Box 3.3). In the more severe reactions, mobilization also occurs of leukotrienes, kinins, and agents precipitating intravascular coagulation.

Intensive bronchospasm, mucosal congestion of the airways with eosinophilic infiltration, and a widespread increase in capillary permeability are the main mechanisms of collapse following an anaphylactic response. Profound arterial and venous dilatation may also occur, with extensive loss of circu-

---

Box 3.2 ● Common agents causing anaphylaxis

- Wasp/Bee stings
- Drugs (penicillin, procainamide, iron compounds, aspirin)
- Foods (nuts, shellfish)
- Blood products, vaccines, hormones, enzymes

Box 3.3 ● Features of anaphylaxis

- Tingling, pruritus, and urticaria
- Nausea, vomiting, and diarrhoea

- Hypotension
- Angio-oedema
- Bronchospasm
- Laryngeal oedema
- Abdominal pain

---

lating fluid into the tissues, a diminished venous return, and a marked fall in systemic arterial pressure. A tachycardia with decreased cardiac output mimicking hypovolaemic shock is common. Less commonly, a paradoxical vagal reaction occurs, with vasodilation and profound cardiac slowing.

Therapy comprises high-flow oxygen, rapid volume expansion with 5 per cent dextrose, and adrenaline. Adrenaline should be given in small aliquots (e.g. 0.1 mg every 2–3 min, intravenously, not subcutaneously, and the dose titrated against the response). Any delay in cannulating a vein in a seriously collapsed patient is an indication for giving the adrenaline intramuscularly. Antihistamine (H_1-antagonists) are commonly given by slow intravenous injection (for example chlorpheniramine 10 mg or diphenhydramine 50 mg). The role of H_2-blocking agents and steroids is more contentious. Intravenous cimetidine has been used with good effect, but experience with this agent is limited; some authors argue against its use. Steroids have no effect in the acute event, but may be considered for bronchospasm and hypotension that is persistent.

If intense bronchospasm and laryngeal oedema, the commonest fatal complications of anaphylaxis, are present, intubate and give urgent treatment with oxygen, intravenous adrenaline, and aminophylline. Consider emergency cricothyroidotomy if an effective airway cannot be established quickly.

Drug overdose and poisoning

A wide variety of agents can threaten tissue oxygenation by their effect on cardiorespiratory function, oxygen transport, or cellular metabolic pathways. The commonest self-poisoning compounds are the minor tranquillizers, the tricyclic antidepressants, and non-narcotic analgesics. Ethanol is also a common drug both of addiction and overdose. Poisoning by narcotic and cardiac drugs is seen frequently. Perhaps surprisingly, the most frequent agent resulting in *fatal* self-poisoning in carbon monoxide from the inhalation of motor-car exhaust fumes.

The majority of episodes of drug overdose are benign, and need only symptomatic treatment together with psychiatric support. In life-threatening cases, unconsciousness with respiratory depression is the most frequent presentation. The mainstay of therapy is therefore attention to the airway and ventilation. Where cardiopulmonary arrest has occurred, full resuscitation will be necessary according to the usual protocols. Note, too, that the patient may be hypothermic.

The nature of the ingested poison should be established as soon as possible so as to minimize danger to medical and nursing staff and to facilitate the planning of further therapy (including active removal of the poison). Specific antidotes to self-poisoning agents are uncommon (Box 3.4), but should be readily available for appropriate cases. Most are safe, and can be given on only a strong suspicion of the nature of the overdose.

Oxygen is an important therapy for carbon monoxide poisoning and in anyone with cardiorespiratory depression. Intravenous glucose and thiamine may be helpful in acute-on-chronic alcohol toxicity. Benzodiazepine poisoning is usually self-limiting with supportive therapy only; but the compound flumazenil (Anexate) may be helpful in severe cases. (Note that flumazenil is not licensed for this use; also, if given to patients overdosed on a mixture of benzodiazepines and tricyclic antidepressants, intractable fitting can occur.)

Tricyclic antidepressants give a miscellany of cardiac arrhythmias, which may be due to their anticholinergic effect, their sympathomimetic action, or their direct depression of myocardial cells and the conducting system. But little pharmacological or electrical help is effective in treating the rhythm disorders associated with tricyclic poisoning. The mainstay of therapy is the correction of acid–base balance with mild alkalinization and by hyperventilation with high levels of inspired oxygen. Prolonged resuscitation attempts have occasionally been successful in tricyclic overdose, particularly in the young or where the patient has become hypothermic before admission.

Box 3.4 ● Antidotes for early use in acute poisoning

Poison	Antidote
Carbon monoxide	Oxygen
Beta blockers	Glucagon 5 mg IV, then 1.5 mg/1 h Dobutamine 500–2000 µg/min
Cyanide	Oxygen, dicobalt edetate 300 mg IV over 3 min Sodium nitrate 10 ml 30% solution IV over 2–4 min
Digoxin	Fab fragments (Digibind) titrated to response
Opioids	Naloxone (Narcan) 0.8–2.0 mg IV repeated every 2–3 min
Benzodiazepines	Flumazenil (Anexate) 200 µg over 125 sec; doses of 100 µg repeated every minute until a satisfactory response is seen or a maximum of 1 mg has been given (usual dose 300–600 µg); but see p. 00.

Box 3.5 gives the telephone numbers of the main UK Poison Centres.

Box 3.5 • Telephone numbers of main UK Poison Centres*

Belfast	01232 240503	Ext. 2140
Birmingham	0121 554 3801	Ext. 5588 or 5589
Cardiff	01222 709901	
Dublin	00353 183 79964	
Edinburgh	0131 536 2300	
Leeds	01132 430715	
	01132 432799	Ext. 3547
London	0171 653 9191	
Newcastle	0191 232 1525	(9 a.m.–5 p.m.)
	0191 232 5131	(After 5 p.m.)

*Correct as at April 1996

Drowning

Anoxia due to submersion is the primary threat to life. Little difference is seen between salt-water and freshwater drowning except that hypernatraemia is a constant feature of immersion in salt-water *if* aspiration or ingestion occurs.

Ten to fifteen per cent of patients develop intense laryngeal spasm, protecting the lungs from aspiration of water or gastric contents ('dry drowning'). The remainder develop pulmonary oedema, which contributes to their continuing hypoxia and acidosis. High alcohol levels, psychotropic agents, hypothermia, silent myocardial infarction, and hypovolaemia due to associated injuries may compound the drowning episode. Hypothermia may prove partially beneficial, however, by affording a degree of cerebral protection, especially in children. Finally, immersion, especially in cold water, may trigger a profound vagal discharge, resulting in cardiac standstill.

The key treatment is effective respiratory support using high levels of inspired oxygen; but head tilt should be avoided because of the frequent association of drowning with injuries to the cervical spine. The early use of atropine may be tried where the heart rate is slow; but circulatory support is best achieved by chest compression, together with attention to oxygenation, core temperature, and the correction of hypovolaemia. The full management of submersion injury is described in the texts cited at the end of this chapter.

Hypothermia

Hypothermia is defined as a core temperature of less than 35 °C, and results in a gradual fall in metabolic rate and oxygen consumption. Predisposing factors are extremes of age, low environmental temperatures, and a reason for immobility (such as stroke, fall, hypothyroidism, alcohol excess, drug overdose, diabetic coma, or exhaustion). Reflex vasoconstriction preserves core temperature, but gives the skin a death-like appearance and makes the pulse extremely difficult to feel. After an initial rise in pulse rate and blood pressure, cardiac output falls, with advancing bradycardia and hypotension. Almost any cardiac arrhythmia can occur in the hypothermic patient; but atrial fibrillation, and then refractory ventricular fibrillation (VF) or asystole are the most common.

Hypothermia calls for aggressive and perhaps prolonged resuscitation, with careful core rewarming. Defibrillation for VF should be applied early, but will often fail while core temperature is low. Cardio-active drugs are usually ineffective, and are best avoided. Open cardiac massage may be indicated, and gives an additional route for cardiac warming.

Resuscitation in late pregnancy

Circulatory arrest from a variety of acute conditions in pregnancy, particularly antepartum haemorrhage remains an important cause of maternal mortality. In the third trimester resuscitation is complicated by compression of the aorta and inferior vena cava (IVC) by the gravid uterus; occlusion of the vena cava in the supine position markedly reduces the chances of successful resuscitation.

Tilting the patient to the left by as little as 30 degrees frees the inferior vena caval blood vessels from compression, but makes resuscitation difficult to perform. Although the resuscitation wedge developed by Rees and Willis may be helpful, the approach currently recommended, in the third trimester, is to perform an emergency Caesarean section if resuscitation has not been successful within 5 minutes. Emergency Caesarean Section—which must be accompanied by uninterrupted cardiopulmonary resuscitation—appears critical to the survival of both mother and baby.

Further reading

1. Austen, K. F. (1987). Disease of immediate type hypersensitivity. In *Harrison's principles of internal medicine*, 11th edn, (ed. J. D. Jeffers, E. J. Scott, and M. Ramos-Englis), pp. 1407–14. McGraw-Hill, New York.
2. Bohn, D. J. (1989). Resuscitation after near drowning and exposure. In *Cardiopulmonary resuscitation*, (ed. P. J. F. Baskett), pp. 195–229. Elsevier, Amsterdam.
3. Consensus development (1980). Thrombolytic therapy in treatment (Summary of an NIH Consensus Conference). *British Medical Journal*, **280**, 1585–7.
4. Danzl, D. F. and Pozos, R. S. (1994). Accidental hypothermia. *New England Journal of Medicine*, **331**, 1756–60.
5. Glassford, D. M., Alford, W. C., Barras, G. R., *et al.* (1981). Pulmonary embolectomy. *Annals of Thoracic Surgery*, **32**, 28–32.
6. Goldhaber, S. Z. (1989). Tissue plasminogen activator in acute pulmonary embolism. *Chest*, **95** (Suppl. Tissue plasminogen activator in cardiopulmonary disease), 281–288S.
7. Harries, M. (1995). Near drowning. In *ABC of resuscitation*, 3rd edn, (ed. M. C. Colquhan, A. J. Handley, and T. R. Evans), pp. 50–3. British Medical Publishing Group, London.
8. Henry, J. A. (1989). Resuscitation from poisoning. In *Cardiopulmonary resuscitation*, (ed. P. J. F. Baskett), pp. 231–57. Elsevier, Amsterdam.
9. Ind, P. W., Causon, R. C., Brown, M. J. and Barnes, P. J. (1985). Circulating catecholamines in acute asthma. *British Medical Journal*, **290**, 267–9.
10. Kelly, J. S. and Prielipp, R. C. (1990). Is cimetidine indicated in the treatment of acute anaphylactic shock? *Anaesthesia and Analgesia*, **71**, 104–5.

11. Kemp, A. M. and Sibert, J. R. (1991). Outcome in children who nearly drown: a British Isles study. *British Medical Journal*, **302**, 931–3.
12. Ledingham, J, G. G. and Weatherall, D. J. (1996). Pulmonary embolism. In *Oxford textbook of medicine*, 3rd edn, (ed. D. J. Weatherall, J. G. G. Ledingham, and D. A. Warrell), pp. 2522–7. Oxford University Press, Oxford.
13. Leeper, K. V., Popovich, J., Lesser, B. A., Adams, D., Froelich, J. W., Burke, M. W., *et al.* (1988). Treatment of massive acute pulmonary embolism. *Chest*, **93**, 234–40.
14. Miller, G. A. H., Sutton, G. C., Kerr, I. H., Gibson, R. V. and Honey, M. (1971). Comparison of streptokinase and heparin in the treatment of isolated acute massive pulmonary embolism. *British Medical Journal*, **2**, 681–4.
15. Oates, S., Williams, G. L. and Rees, G. A. D. (1988). Cardiopulmonary resuscitation in late pregnancy. *British Medical Journal*, **297**, 404–5.
16. *Oxford textbook of medicine*, 3rd edn, (ed. D. J. Weatherall, J. G. G. Ledingham, and D. A. Warrell), Chapter 13, pp. 356–60. Oxford University Press, Oxford.
17. Parke, T. R. J., Steedman, D. J., Robertson, C. E., Little, R. A. and Maycock, P. F. (1992). Plasma catecholamine responses in severe asthma. *Archives of Emergency Medicine*, **9**, 157–61
18. Rees, G. A. D. and Willis, B. A. (1988). Resuscitation in late pregnancy. *Anaesthesia*, **43**, 347–9.
19. Seaton, A., Seaton, D. and Leitch, A. G. (1989). Pulmonary embolism. In *Crofton and Douglas' respiratory disease*, (4th edn), pp. 539–66. Blackwell, London.
20. Senior, R. (1988). Pulmonary embolism. In *Cecil textbook of medicine*, (18th edn, ed. J. B. Wyngaarden and L. H. Smith), pp. 442–50. Saunders, Philadelphia.
21. de Soto, H. and Turk, P. (1989). Cimetidine in anaphylactic shock refractory to standard therapy. *Anaesthesia and Analgesia*, **69**, 264–5.
22. Steedman, D. (1994). *Environmental emergencies*. Oxford University Press.
23. Stuart Taylor, M. E. (1990). Management of near drowning. *Hospital Update*, **May**, 419–31.
24. Whitman, J. G. (1991). Flumazenil. *Prescriber's Journal*, **31**, 57–61.

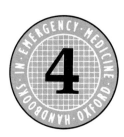

CHAPTER 4

Resuscitation in hospital

Key points in resuscitation in hospital

1 Successful resuscitation in hospital depends on organization and training as well as on the use of agreed protocols for optimum therapy.

2 A commitment by consultants and senior nursing staff to support the resuscitation service is vital.

3 A multidisciplinary Resuscitation Committee should meet regularly to promote widespread interest in resuscitation, to establish hospital-wide standards, to review equipment needs and developments, and to audit the practicalities and outcomes of resuscitation attempts.

4 Training in resuscitation is the primary responsibility of a designated Resuscitation Training Officer, who should arrange tuition, accreditation, and team practices for all relevant staff. The role should include the audit of arrest procedures and general oversight of all resuscitation equipment.

5 Equipment for resuscitation should be clearly identified, regularly checked, and readily available—particularly devices for basic life support and the defibrillator/monitor.

6 The 'crash-call-out' system should be familiar to all staff, and should be tested at the beginning of each shift.

7 Staff in the Accident and Emergency Department, Cardiac Care Unit, and Intensive Care Unit must be competent in resuscitation, as well as being able to draw on the hospital crash team when necessary.

8 Training senior nurses to defibrillate should be considered for areas of particularly high dependency.

9 Remember the needs of relatives when a resuscitation attempt has been completed, particularly if it was unsuccessful.

Introduction

In addition to medical skills, efficient resuscitation in hospital requires careful organization. This chapter addresses some of the practicalities of running a hospital resuscitation service, beginning with the general requirements for organization, training, and equipment. In several areas of the hospital (e.g. A&E, the CCU, and the ICU) the availability of equipment and staff will be different from that regularly provided by the hospital crash team; these areas need to develop specific plans for the best management of their patients.

Organization

The key to developing a successful resuscitation service is that a specific interest and responsibility for this provision is taken up by senior medical and nursing personnel. The effective management of a cardiac arrest requires team work, and the organization of a resuscitation service should also be focused on a team approach.

A multidisciplinary Resuscitation Committee should be established (Box 4.1), and should meet regularly. The importance of including senior staff cannot be over-emphasized, and representation of those who regularly manage cardiac arrests is mandatory. Other staff can be seconded either as permanent members or for special discussions. These might include porters, telephonists, pharmacists, or ambulance personnel.

The main tasks of the Committee are listed in Box 4.2. It will need to consider in detail all the practicalities of providing an efficient response to cardiac arrest, as well as the more general issue of raising the (often far from prominent) profile of resuscitation as a vital medical activity. It should also be conscious of the need to evaluate and introduce new technology and techniques, and to provide agreed guidelines on the logistics of communicating a decision of 'not for resuscitation' to those involved when an arrest occurs.

Box 4.1 ● Suggested membership of a Hospital Resuscitation Committee

- A leading consultant
  with a specific interest in resuscitation
- Consultant representatives
  from general medicine, cardiology, general surgery, anaesthetics/intensive care, accident and emergency
- Senior nursing staff
  including those working in high-dependency areas
- Resuscitation Training Officer
- Representative(s) of junior medical staff participating in crash teams

---

Box 4.2 ● The tasks of a Hospital Resuscitation Committee

- To raise general awareness of the need for a highly organized response to the collapsed patient
- To enhance liaison between key personnel in matters of resuscitation
- To promote and monitor resuscitation training and certification for junior medical and nursing staff
- To oversee the provision, maintenance, and standardization of resuscitation equipment
- To effect changes in service provision and training that will improve the practice of resuscitation
- To audit all aspects of arrest procedures
- To provide for the hospital community regular data reviewing the incidence, location, nature, and outcome of attempted resuscitations in hospital

---

Training and the role of the Resuscitation Training Officer

All members of a resuscitation team must be trained adequately in the various skills that they will require at a cardiac

---

Box 4.3 • Suggested equipment for resuscitation training in hospital

Hands-on equipment

Essential

- Arrhythmia/defibrillation torso with pulse generator, printer, ECG simulator, VF recognition module
- Skillmeter resuscitation torso (adult)
- Baby model
- Adult intubation trainer
- Infusion trainer

Optional

- Additional ECG simulator interface
–junior model
–infant intubation trainer

General equipment

- Video replay machine with TV/monitor
- Computer/printer/database software (for record keeping)
- Projector and screen
- Cleaning equipment with nearby running water

---

arrest. We recommend that medical staff should be trained in advanced life support (ALS) to the standards laid down by the Resuscitation Council (UK).

Training is a time-consuming task. In practice, it is best supervised by a designated Resuscitation Training Officer (RTO) who has access to adequate space and aids for teaching. (Box 4.3 lists suggested training equipment.) The RTO—whose background may be in nursing, the ambulance service, or the technical grades—will be responsible throughout the hospital for initial and refresher training in both the theory and practice of resuscitation. Two benefits accrue: first, that staff are trained and accredited in basic and advanced life-support; and secondly, that those being trained will learn protocols that are uniform throughout the organization. These protocols should be based on the guidelines of the Resuscitation Council (UK) (inside back cover). Their existence will ensure that members of the cardiac arrest team have similar expectations of the way an arrest will be managed, including their expectations as to the distribution of responsibilities among team members.

Team-based practices in resuscitation, using mannikins which simulate cardiac arrhythmias and can be defibrillated, are essential. The location of 'mock arrests' can be varied throughout the hospital to mimic everyday experiences. No other form of training gives experience in the team leadership and co-ordination required for an efficient resuscitation attempt. The RTO should arrange and supervise such simulated arrests, giving educational feedback and ensuring regular participation by all relevant staff. Team practices can also lead to the formation of a well co-ordinated demonstration group that can be used for instruction and for increasing awareness of resuscitation procedures.

Box 4.4 ● The role of the Resuscitation Training Officer

- Co-ordinate and supervise resuscitation training throughout the hospital
- Arrange appropriate tests for accreditation
- Organize regular team practices of managing a simulated cardiac arrest
- Oversee regular checking procedures for resuscitation equipment
- Stimulate an interest in resuscitation activities
- Collect and present data auditing the resuscitation service.
- Liaise with the Resuscitation Committee, other professional groups, and all staff involved with the practicalities of resuscitation in hospital
- Provide advice on resuscitation as necessary

The RTO will also provide a source of advice on resuscitation and a general overview of the location, care, and performance of the equipment, offering suggestions on how it should be replaced or improved. He or she should be able to supply data relating to resuscitation attempts throughout the hospital, including patient profiles, the clinical presentation of arrests, personnel involved, treatment given, outcome, and observations on performance. The role of the Resuscitation Training Officer is summarized in Box 4.4.

Equipment

The equipment for managing cardiopulmonary arrest in hospital should be easily accessible. Standardized kits for basic life support should be clearly identified and available immediately in all wards and other areas of busy clinical activity. The responsibility for ensuring that these kits are in place and checked regularly should be allocated unambiguously to a senior member of the nursing (or perhaps the technical) staff working in the area.

A similar arrangement should apply to the defibrillators, monitors, trolleys, and boxes used for advanced life support. These will be fewer, being placed in high-dependency units and within easy reach of, though not necessarily present in, all main patient areas. The degree to which different pieces of ALS equipment are kept together will vary from hospital to hospital; but the number of items to move from place to place should be minimized. Special emphasis should be given to providing ready access to defibrillator/monitors and to devices for airway management. Hospital-wide standardization of defibrillator/monitors will ensure operator familiarity when time is at a premium. A system whereby restocked kits are sealed until use together with an efficient system of checking and replacement after use gives arrest teams confidence that they will find all they need in the heat of the moment.

All health care professionals should know the location of equipment for basic and advanced life support in the vicinity of their usual work. But this ideal is rarely achieved; all too often such knowledge is gathered hurriedly in a desperate search for essential items when a patient has collapsed. It should be taught during an induction period, and again at subsequent resuscitation training.

Staff working in any clinical area should be aware of the

location and operation of drip stands, power points (with plugs that fit), local emergency call buttons, and the 'crash call' number operated by the hospital telephone system. This should be a unique and well-known code easily visible on every phone. The ideal of a universal alert number throughout all UK hospitals would clearly be worth while, but has yet to be achieved. (Checking the call-out system is discussed on p. 54.)

Specific areas

Accident and Emergency Department

The Accident and Emergency Department must be well-prepared for the management of patients suffering cardiopulmonary arrest as it is, regrettably, a common occurrence. It may arise as a result of medical, surgical, or traumatic conditions; but the guidance given in this chapter will concentrate on the commonest of these—the 'medical' cardiac arrest.

Patients may be presented by the ambulance service, having arrested *en route* to hospital or, more commonly, having been discovered in an already-collapsed state. Advance warning of the arrival of a collapsed patient in A&E should be available by radio or telephone link from ambulance control. This will allow adequate arrangements to be made for the patient's reception, including the provision of a trolley, porters, and the resuscitation team. All patients brought in this way should be assessed in the light and space of the A&E Department; it is not acceptable to rely only on a brief assessment in a darkened ambulance to decide whether to continue or abandon resuscitation.

Not infrequently, patients arrest while in the A&E Department itself, usually during the course of a myocardial infarction, but occasionally from respiratory causes such as acute severe asthma. Given the frequency of cardiac arrests—about a hundred for every fifty thousand patients seen per year—the A&E Department must be supplied with a well-lit, adequately sized resuscitation room with two or more treatment bays (Fig. 4.1).

The equipment necessary for resuscitation must be of high quality, comparatively easy to use, reliable, and robust. The basic requirements are as follows:

(1) a trolley-mounted monitor/defibrillator;
(2) patient trolleys with a head-down facility, robust enough for patient transfer to other areas of the hospital;
(3) airway management and ventilation equipment; and
(4) equipment for peripheral and central venous cannulation.

Although senior A&E staff often conduct resuscitation attempts themselves, few accident departments in the United Kingdom have senior A&E staff on site 24 hours a day; the hospital crash team will therefore be required to attend A&E cardiac arrests when senior A&E staff are not available.

The A&E Department crash team will usually comprise:

- A&E Consultant;
- A&E Senior Registrar/Registrar;
- A&E Senior House Officer; and
- two nurses from the A&E Department.

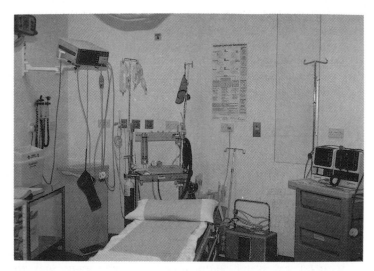

Fig. 4.1 • A treatment bay in the resuscitation room at St. Bartholomew's Hospital, showing the equipment required for a resuscitation attempt.

The hospital crash team will ideally consist of:

- Resuscitation Registrar (an Anaesthetic Senior Registrar/Registrar, often also covering intensive care);
- General Physician (Registrar/Senior Registrar);
- House Physician; and
- two nurses from the area where the arrest occurs.

Each team will require a team leader, who may be either the Physician or the Resuscitation Registrar in the hospital crash team, but will be the A&E Consultant in the A&E team.

The attendance of the personnel listed above underlines the value of having senior staff taking part in a resuscitation attempt. If local staffing arrangements do not allow these suggested patterns, maintain the principle of including staff in the crash team who are as experienced as possible.

Dual cover for arrests in A&E is useful. Whereas the hospital crash team will be available throughout the 24-hour period, individuals on that team are usually busy, either in high-dependency units or in servicing acute medical admissions. The skills necessary for cardiopulmonary resuscitation are well within the scope of A&E staff, and a department-based system allows the development of a close-knit team approach, as well as sharply defining A&E's policies for resuscitation. It also allows for the all-important post-arrest review, usually conducted by the senior member of staff involved, which gives an opportunity for immediate feedback, leading, if necessary, to improvements in team performance. The review will also offer an invaluable forum for doctors and nurses to express any anxieties felt during the resuscitation that might never otherwise come to light.

The call-out system for both A&E and hospital crash teams must work faultlessly. It should be checked at the beginning of each shift. Any team member not responding to the test must be bleeped repeatedly until he or she acknowledges the call. Failing this, a replacement must be found urgently. The absence of a key team member at a cardiac arrest not only seriously affects the management of the patient, but is also distressing for other team members, who may feel that the outcome could have been different had the missing team member been present.

One of the particular problems of attempted resuscitation in

A&E is that the immediate events surrounding the cardiac arrest are often unknown to the team. Even basic information, such as the age of the patient and length of the cardiopulmonary standstill, may be unavailable. Hence resuscitation may be commenced on patients who, in retrospect, were unlikely to benefit from such an attempt. But this is preferable to failing to resuscitate patients who are subsequently discovered to have had a good chance of survival. In general, therefore, when a cardiac arrest team is presented with a patient who has suffered a cardiopulmonary arrest, resuscitation should begin while further information is being gathered.

Information about the patient may be available from ambulance personnel, and possibly from relatives who have accompanied the patient to hospital. Relatives should initially be taken by a senior member of staff to a designated room in a quiet area of the department. The room should be pleasantly decorated and equipped with a telephone from which outside calls can be made. There should be at least four comfortable chairs and a small table.

A senior nurse should remain with the relatives at all times until either the patient is transferred to a ward or all the formalities have been completed if the patient has died. Usually, neither the nurse nor any other member of the team will know the patient or the relatives. It is sensible in these circumstances to give reassurance to the effect that all possible efforts are being made to save the patient, but that his or her condition is serious. Relatives should be reassured that they will be told immediately of any information that becomes available. Enquiries should be made about any other relatives who may need to be contacted—but actual contact should be delayed until the final outcome is known. Specific questions should be asked about any religious beliefs held by the patient or relatives. These may call for ministers of religion to be contacted or other arrangements to be made.

Patients successfully resuscitated should be transferred promptly either to the Cardiac Care (CCU) or to the Intensive Care Unit (ICU), depending on the need for continued ventilation. A short time after this the relatives should be accompanied to the appropriate ward and introduced to the senior nursing staff there. Details of the information already given to the relatives should be relayed clearly on handover to the ward staff. Relatives should be given a contact phone number and reassured that if they wish to know more about what happened in the A&E Department they can use this number to ring the Consultant.

If the patient in A&E dies, then this fact must be relayed clearly to the relatives as soon as death has been confirmed. Various formalities must be complied with and the family should be asked whether they wish to see their relative in the resuscitation room or the hospital's Chapel of Rest. There is usually a hospital steward who will deal with the formal requirements in a sympathetic fashion. Further details of how to handle this situation are discussed in Chapter 10.

Cardiac and Intensive Care Units

In these high-dependency areas, patients are inevitably at increased risk of malignant arrhythmias, and cardiac monitoring will be universal. Many patients on the ICU will be receiving intensive cardiopulmonary support, with mechanical ventilation, inotropes, and perhaps temporary cardiac pacing. Patients will be under close observation by the nursing staff, in addition to being connected to a variety of automatic alarms. Medical staff are often close at hand.

In spite of this intense supervision, delays in responding to an abrupt loss of cardiac output may be surprisingly long. Electromechanical dissociation and even major arrhythmias may initially go unnoticed; the close monitoring of these units is no guarantee of a rapid response to collapse. There can be a disturbing tendency for nursing and medical staff to act solely on the basis of monitor traces or alarms, and to neglect the clinical state of the patient.

In the Cardiac Care Unit all major causes of circulatory arrest—ventricular fibrillation/rapid ventricular tachycardia, asystole, and electromechanical dissociation—will be seen commonly, and will often occur without warning. In patients with acute myocardial infarction, ventricular fibrillation usually develops soon after admission, whether or not thrombolytic therapy has been given. If initial left ventricular function is good, rapid defibrillation according to the recommended protocol (p. 20) is likely to be both effective and worthwhile. It is therefore mandatory that the nursing staff are trained, accredited, and provided with equipment to defibrillate with minimal delay and without the need to wait for the arrival of the crash team.

Ventricular fibrillation may also occur as the final irreversible event in progressive deterioration from cardiogenic shock. In these patients it should be clear ahead of time whether a resuscitation attempt is appropriate or not. But it should also be emphasized that a decision against resuscitation is not synonymous with abandoning all hope for recovery through continuing intensive care.

Intensive and Cardiac Care Units should carry a wide range of readily available cardioactive drugs for use in cardiovascular emergencies. For example, it should be possible rapidly to provide injections/infusions of lignocaine, atropine, adrenaline, isoprenaline, inotropes, amiodarone, digoxin, and nitrates. Second- and third-line anti-arrhythmic drugs (see p. 133) should be within easy reach.

Specialist equipment for advanced life support should also be available, including devices for external pacing and pericardial aspiration. Facilities for temporary transvenous pacing should be ready for immediate use, ideally using X-ray screening for the insertion of the wire. Ventricular demand pacing should be available at a variety of rates via a lead configuration that is unipolar (for acute myocardial ischaemia/infarction) or bipolar (for conducting system disease). Additional facilities and expertise for atrial pacing, 'overdrive' pacing for ventricular tachycardia, and AV sequential and AV synchronous pacing will give a greater range of therapeutic options, but are likely to be less widely available.

Although the CCU and the ICU may be well equipped for respiratory and circulatory support, it is essential that the materials and equipment necessary to deal with cardiac arrest are kept together, readily available, mobile, and in a location well known to all who work on the unit. They should be checked at the beginning of every shift, and back-up material should be available for immediate substitution when required.

The general ward

Resuscitation attempts frequently occur within the main hospital, but relatively infrequently on any one particular ward.

This means that individual wards require clear protocols for calling the crash team, as well as regular refresher training regarding equipment, drugs, etc.

The Resuscitation Committee should encourage all Consultants responsible for in-patients to decide whether or not individual patients are to be resuscitated. The information should be given unambiguously to the nursing staff by the Consultant in charge of the patient. Some form of indication in the nursing records is essential to ensure that resuscitation attempts are not initiated inappropriately. Thus, a junior nurse left alone in charge of a ward full of patients should be in no doubt as to when to call the crash team.

In the event of a cardiac arrest, basic life support should commence pending the arrival of the team. This will usually be restricted to external chest compression and mouth-to-mask ventilation. Curtains or screens should be drawn around the bed, and one nurse should be made available to reassure other patients on the ward.

Depending on the construction of the bed, a bed board may be needed, or the patient may need to be transferred to the floor. On the arrival of the crash team the team leader should be identified to the senior nurse present, in order to avoid confusion. The senior nurse must be constantly available to ensure the provision of equipment and drugs as and when they are requested; but the scene should not become overcrowded with non-participating onlookers.

Depending on the outcome, the patient may need transfer to the Cardiac Care or Intensive Care Unit; but in any event the relatives should be informed at the earliest opportunity. Before the crash team departs, the team leader should speak to the relatives in person. It is rarely sensible to explain such an event over the telephone—it is sufficient to say that the patient has deteriorated rapidly and that the relatives should come to the hospital immediately.

Further reading

1. Gordon, C. and Newman, B. (1989). Resuscitation in hospitals. In *Cardiopulmonary resuscitation*, (ed. P. J. F. Baskett), pp. 385–97. Elsevier, Amsterdam.

2. Kaye, W., Mancini, M. E., Rallis, S. F. and Wynne, G. (1989). Training and evaluation in basic and advanced resuscitation. In *Cardiopulmonary resuscitation*, (ed. P. J. F. Baskett), pp. 314–45. Elsevier, Amsterdam.
3. Royal College of Physicians (1987). Resuscitation from cardiopulmonary arrest. Training and organisation. *Journal of the Royal College of Physicians*, **21**, 1–8.
4. Seraj, M. A. and Naguib, M. (1990). Cardiopulmonary resuscitation skills of medical professionals. *Resuscitation*, **20**, 31–9.

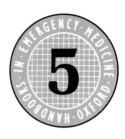

CHAPTER 5

Management of myocardial infarction

Key points in the management of acute myocardial infarction

1 Acute myocardial infarction usually results from abrupt occlusion of a coronary artery by a combination of thrombosis and spasm. Myocardial damage follows swiftly resulting in mechanical failure and electrical instability. Enhanced autonomic tone aggravates this unstable situation.

2 Diagnosis rests primarily on a characteristic history supplemented by an ECG showing ST elevation. Other ECG changes compatible with infarction (including left-bundle branch-block, marked ST segment depression, and steep T wave inversion) should be interpreted in the light of the history and examination.

3 Myocardial infarction should be treated as soon as possible after the onset of symptoms. The first few hours of an attack are associated with the highest risk of ventricular fibrillation—and with the greatest chance of reopening the occluded coronary artery by thrombolysis.

4 Initial treatment should comprise reassurance, sublingual nitrate, oxygen, and pain relief using intravenous opioids with an anti-emetic.

5 Thrombolytic therapy and aspirin should be given to all patients with definite acute myocardial infarction provided there are no risks of allergy or serious haemorrhage.

6 Intravenous nitrates, beta blockers, and ACE inhibitors have favourable effects in specific patient groups.

7 Routine anti-arrhythmic treatment (e.g. lignocaine) is not recommended.

8 Heparin is often advised: in low dose subcutaneously for those who have received thrombolytic therapy, and at full dose intravenously for those who have not.

9 Heart failure requires early and aggressive treatment, using oxygen and intravenous opioids, anti-emetics, nitrates, and diuretics. Consider the use of digoxin in those with alveolar oedema. The diabetic patient and those on previous oral beta blocking drugs are at special risk of this complication.

Introduction

Unstable coronary syndromes, particularly acute myocardial infarction, so often cause cardiac arrest that to consider their management is essential. A substantial reduction in mortality from heart attack can now be achieved not only from successful resuscitation, but on a wider scale by appropriate treatment with iv opioids, aspirin, nitrates, beta blockers, thrombolytic agents, ACE inhibitors, and anticoagulants. How these agents exert their beneficial effect is becoming clearer as we understand more of the pathological mechanisms of acute coronary occlusion and its resulting effect on the myocardium.

Pathology of acute myocardial infarction

Myocardial infarction usually results from abrupt occlusion of a coronary artery. The subsequent response of the heart muscle and systemic factors also influence the final outcome of this rapidly evolving syndrome.

Mechanisms of coronary occlusion

Almost always, acute coronary narrowing occurs at a site of pre-existing atheroma. Often the atheromatous deposit has been too small to exert any noticeable effect on myocardial perfusion, and the existence of coronary disease is announced only with the acute event.

The distorted form of an atheromatous lesion predisposes to plaque rupture or haemorrhage, events that trigger a cascading process culminating in coronary occlusion (Fig. 5.1). Platelet activation by disrupted endothelium initiates the formation of intraluminal clot, and in addition releases substances that cause marked vasoconstriction. If intraplaque haemorrhage occurs, the coronary lesion expands, reducing further the luminal diameter. In addition, plaque rupture induces inflammation in the adventitia of the artery, and this also predisposes to spasm.

Intraluminal thrombosis is responsible for the majority of episodes of acute coronary occlusion resulting in unstable angina or myocardial infarction. But in as many as 25 per cent of cases plaque haemorrhage or intense spasm predominate. (Thrombolytic therapy in such patients will be of little help.)

The process of coronary thrombosis is dynamic. It involves fluctuating vascular tone and a variable balance between clot formation and lysis through simultaneous activation of both fibrinogen and plasminogen pathways (Fig. 5.2). A single major occlusive event may be heralded by a brief stuttering pattern of narrowing, giving rise to attacks of 'warning' coronary pain at rest. Less commonly, there is intermittent coronary narrowing, with episodes of rest pain, over several days. In these cases careful management is necessary to avoid progression to a completed infarct, though this may occur even with optimal therapy in hospital.

Mention must also be made of the small platelet thrombi that can develop on the roughened surface of an atheromatous plaque. Though they pose no threat to coronary flow, they can

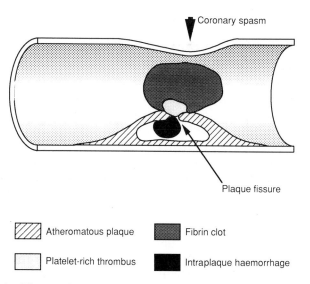

Fig. 5.1 • The mechanism of acute coronary occlusion, including plaque rupture, intraplaque haemorrhage, platelet activation, intraluminal clot, and coronary spasm.

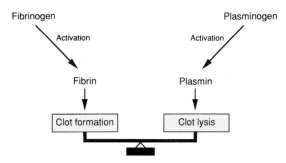

Fig. 5.2 • The balance between the fibrinogen and plasminogen systems.

embolize to the distal coronary tree, creating small, patchy areas of profound ischaemia and marked electrical instability. Therein lies an important and common mechanism for sudden cardiac death, associated with atheromatous but patent arteries and no macroscopic infarction.

The myocardium

The myocardium downstream from an occluded coronary vessel suffers rapidly from a deprivation of oxygen and glucose. Muscle relaxation is affected first (in under a minute), stiffening the ischaemic area; contraction failure of the threatened segment follows swiftly, though this is often countered by hyperactivity of the remaining myocardial wall.

In addition to these mechanical effects, electrical instability is the hallmark of an evolving infarct. Differential recovery times of adjacent myocardial cells and re-entry through small amounts of damaged, slowly conducting tissue (see p. 165) predispose to ventricular tachycardia and fibrillation.

Myocardial necrosis begins early—perhaps within 5 minutes—and is usually complete in 30–60 minutes. Cellular swelling, mitochondrial breakdown, leucocyte activation, a local increase in catecholamines, and the rapid accumulation of intracellular calcium contribute to this speedy demise.

Systemic effects

The dynamic process of myocardial infarction is adversely affected by a systemic neurohumoral response. A rise in circulating catecholamines increases myocardial workload by its effect on heart rate and blood-pressure, and additionally predisposes to malignant tachyarrhythmias. Simultaneous activation of the parasympathetic system, causing a marked autonomic imbalance, makes ventricular fibrillation even more likely. If vagal tone predominates, sinus bradycardia and AV nodal block are likely, perhaps associated with hypotension and 'escape' ventricular arrhythmias.

Diagnosis

Symptoms

The clinical presentation of myocardial infarction is usually straightforward. Cardiac pain is commonly described as 'a pressure', 'squeezing', 'an ache', 'tightness', or as 'a weight on the chest'; and many patients are convinced that they are suffering from indigestion. Pain is never sharp, pleuritic, or stabbing, nor does it begin instantaneously. (Such sudden pain suggests aortic dissection.)

Inferior infarction may be represented by pain that extends into the epigastrium; but radiation to the back is rare. A similarity to previous angina is helpful, patients usually noting that their pain has become more intense, is occurring at rest, and has not been relieved by GTN. But comparison with previous symptoms may be unreliable, particularly in patients who have received coronary surgery. Also, diabetic patients appear to suffer less pain (and more heart failure) than non-diabetics; and for those presenting in pulmonary oedema, breathlessness may be the overriding symptom.

The pain of an infarct has a disagreeable quality, and is often, but not inevitably, accompanied by sweating and nausea. Continuous, prolonged pain (perhaps for more than 4 hours) is more likely to represent unstable angina than true infarction. (Muscle needs to be alive to hurt!)

Signs

In acute myocardial infarction physical signs are common but may be subtle. The effects of sympathetic over-activity—pallor, sweating, and an anxious expression—will be obvious. Changes in blood pressure and heart rate may be noted. Other findings require more careful observation: a palpable area of dyskinetic ventricular movement (a systolic bulging to the left of the sternum) and an additional third or fourth heart sound are common in anterior infarction; a bradycardia and a raised venous pressure (from right ventricular dysfunction) are frequent signs in an inferior infarct.

The electrocardiogram

The electrocardiogram of the 'classic' myocardial infarction is easy to recognize: Q waves, ST segment elevation, and T wave inversion are characteristic (Fig. 5.3). But recent emphasis on a rapid response to patients with acute infarction has drawn attention to the more subtle ECG patterns of its 'hyperacute' phase. Here, broad T waves with no identifiable ST–T wave junction, and early straight or concave-upward ST segment elevation are typical (Fig. 5.4). Differentiation from a physiological high take-off pattern can be difficult, although the clinical context will help, and serial ECGs (the first being repeated in 20–30 minutes) may clarify the diagnosis. An evolving inferior infarct can be confirmed by the often associated ST segment depression in leads I and aVL or in the anteroseptal leads (Fig. 5.5).

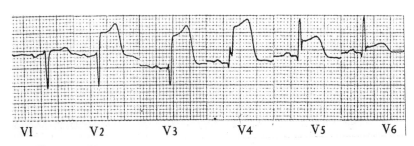

VI   V2   V3   V4   V5   V6

Fig. 5.3 ●Characteristic electrocardiogram of acute myocardial infarction, showing early Q waves and marked ST segment elevation.

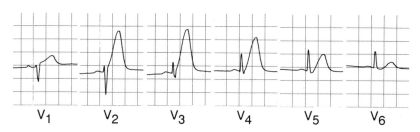

Fig. 5.4 ● The more subtle ST–T changes of a 'hyperacute' infarct.

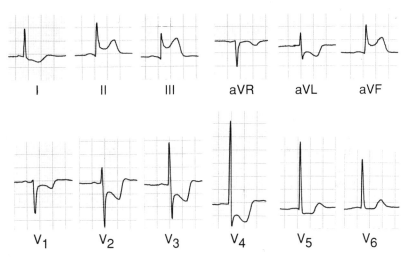

Fig. 5.5 ● The injury current (ST elevation) of an inferior infarction is shown in leads II, III, and aVF associated with marked ST depression in the lateral leads (I, aVL), and anteroseptal leads (V$_1$–V$_4$).

Occasionally, a myocardial infarct is associated with non-specific ST–T changes or profound ST depression only. A left-bundle branch-block pattern is always abnormal, but is usually considered 'non-diagnostic' for infarction unless 'unexpected' ST elevation is seen (Fig. 5.6).

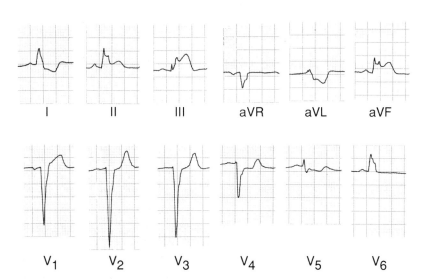

Fig. 5.6 • Left-bundle branch-block associated with unusual ST segment elevation in leads II and III, and aVF indicating an acute inferior infarction.

Biochemical markers of necrosis ('cardiac enzymes')

Necrosing myocardial cells release a variety of compounds into the perfusing blood although washout into the peripheral circulation forms only a small fraction (<10 per cent) of the locally released activity. The ideal biochemical marker would rise within an hour, remain elevated for several days, be entirely specific for myocardial tissue, and faithfully represent the extent of myocardial necrosis. No current marker lives up to these ideals. The best-known compound is creatine kinase (CK) and its more specific myocardial fraction CK-MB. In as many as 25 per cent of patients, CK activity rises within 1 hour of the onset of major symptoms; but it gives a positive test in only just over 50 per cent of cases by 4 hours, rising to about 80 per cent at 6 hours. A protein marker of more recent interest is myoglobin, although it shares with CK a lack of specificity for myocardial tissue. Myoglobin rises more quickly than CK—89 per cent positive at 4 hours—but its peak at 8–12 hours is short-lived.

The value of myoglobin, CK, and CK-MB estimated on admission by a near-patient analyser for cases of suspected myocardial infarction was investigated recently by Lee and colleagues. It appeared that in the early hours of an infarct the ECG remained the more valuable diagnostic tool with little additional contribution from these biochemical markers.

New indicators of myocardial damage—troponin T, I, and C (components of the contractile protein) invite interest because of their very high specificity for heart muscle. But the time-course of appearance of troponin is similar to that of CK-MB limiting its use for the confirmation of an infarct within the first few hours.

Urgent enzyme estimations—even with on-site analysis—seem to play a limited role in the early diagnosis of acute myocardial infarction. A negative result even up to 6 hours is no guarantee against the occurrence of an infarct. Moreover, the value of the thrombolytic therapy for patients with an early CK rise where the ECG and/or history is equivocal has not yet been demonstrated.

Routine treatment

Aims and initial management

The first aim of treatment is to relieve pain, and the second is to preserve life by correcting and preventing major arrhythmias. The third aim is to preserve viable myocardium—by reducing ventricular workload and by restoring coronary blood flow. Ideally, this should occur while jeopardized cells still have the potential for recovery; but benefit seems to accrue from relatively late reopening of the vessel, either by thrombolytic agents or (rarely) by mechanical intervention.

Initial management begins by offering calm reassurance and placing the patient in a position of maximum comfort. This will usually be sitting up, unless cerebral perfusion is severely compromised, when the patient will appreciate being more horizontal. Leg elevation is never required.

Oxygen

Even in an uncomplicated infarct, ventilation—perfusion mismatch predisposes to hypoxaemia. For those with clinical or radiological evidence of left-heart failure supplemental oxygen is mandatory. Some patients find a conventional mask claustrophobic; in these cases—particularly if it is unnecessary to provide a high concentration of oxygen—consider the use of nasal speculae.

Analgesia

The pain of acute myocardial infarction is due to the continuing intense ischaemia of living but jeopardized myocardium. It signals not only suffering for the patient but heart muscle at risk, and a state of autonomic imbalance that predisposes to shock and fatal arrhythmias. Relieving the pain and distress of an evolving infarct is therefore an urgent priority. In the long term, therapies to reduce continuing ischaemia—including nitrates and thrombolytics—will prove the most beneficial. But the immediate use of iv opioid analgesics is mandatory unless the patient is calm and virtually pain-free on presentation.

We use diamorphine 5 mg given intravenously at a rate of 1 mg/min titrated to the patient's response. (This will seem slow—and it should!) Further increments of 2.5 mg at 10-minute intervals are recommended until pain relief is achieved. The first dose should be 2.5 mg for small or elderly patients, for those who have already received analgesia, and for patients with chronic respiratory disease. (Naloxone should always be to hand if sensitivity to opioid is suspected.)

Opioids must be given with an anti-emetic, since they so often cause nausea of a 'motion sickness' type. (Imprudent handling of the patient during transport by trolley will aggravate this.) Cyclizine is a convenient drug, as it can be used to dissolve diamorphine crystals for combined administration. Give 50 mg cyclizine for every 5 mg diamorphine. Cyclizine is contraindicated in severe left ventricular failure or cardiogenic shock because of its constricting effect on peripheral coronary end arterioles. Metoclopramide is a suitable alternative, but cannot be used to dissolve the opioid.

Hypotension may follow opioid administration, but is usually short-lived, and may be partially reversed by naloxone. If it is associated with bradycardia, lay the patient flat. Atropine 300–600 μg intravenously will usually be helpful.

Nitrates

Nitrates have a beneficial haemodynamic effect in acute ischaemic syndromes—including myocardial infarction—through three sites of action: the coronary arteries, the venous capacitance vessels, and the peripheral arterioles.

In the coronary arteries, nitrates appear to mimic the action of the naturally occurring endothelial relaxation factor, nitric oxide. The effect of nitrates on the abnormal coronary constriction associated with a ruptured atheromatous plaque, or on 'pure' spasm, is variable, but may be marked and therefore valuable.

Venodilatation by nitrates reduces the return of blood to the heart (its 'pre-load'). The consequent reduction in ventricular filling pressure and heart size lessens myocardial oxygen requirement at a time when coronary flow is in jeopardy. A reduction in peripheral arterial tone further reduces myocardial workload by reducing the resistance to blood flow presented to the heart (the 'after-load').

Although regular oral nitrates after acute myocardial infarction seem to produce no overall benefit, the early use of sublingual or buccal nitrate is worthwhile for pain relief, provided that the blood pressure is not unduly low. The cautious use of intravenous nitrates may still be valuable in patients with continuing pain or radiographic evidence of heart failure. An appropriate schedule would be glyceryl trinitrate 12.5–100 microgram/min, titrated so that the heart rate does not exceed 100 per minute or the systolic blood pressure fall below 100 mmHg.

Aspirin

An important reduction in mortality is observed when aspirin is used up to 24 hours after the onset of major symptoms. Aspirin's beneficial effect has been confirmed both for unstable angina and acute myocardial infarction (Fig. 5.7), but the mechanisms involved are unclear. The prevention of clot extension, a reduction in platelet 'stickiness' to improve capil-

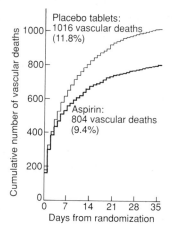

Fig. 5.7 ● The benefit in mortality from the use of aspirin in myocardial infarction.

lary flow, and perhaps a lessening of the inflammatory response both at the site of plaque rupture and in the infarcted area may all contribute to aspirin's beneficial effect. Recent studies show that aspirin may exert its beneficial effect chiefly through reducing the chances of re-occlusion.

No clear guidelines exist for the best dose, but the use of 300 mg per day for the first day, and then 75 mg daily is likely to obtain the required therapeutic effect. Aspirin should be given as soon as *practicable* after the onset of major symptoms—but there is no need for panic! Relief of pain and nausea/vomiting take higher priority. A chewable tablet will be absorbed more rapidly than one swallowed but neither will be helpful in a patient who is distressed or vomiting.

Thrombolytic therapy

In the past ten years coronary thrombolysis has moved centre-stage in the management of myocardial infarction. Its impact for preserving heart muscle and reducing mortality has proved one of the most dramatic advances of the decade.

Mechanism of action Thrombolytic agents activate plasminogen to form the specific fibrin-digesting protein, plasmin. Plasminogen is a normal component of circulating blood, and also binds strongly to fibrin wherever it is formed. The activation of clot-bound plasminogen results in progressive clot lysis; the activation of circulating plasminogen may degrade circulatory fibrinogen ('fibrinogenolysis'), leading to a systemic lytic state in which blood clotting throughout the body is depressed. Thrombolytic agents may act equally on circulating and bound plasminogen, or may show a relatively high affinity for bound fibrin, making them 'clot-specific'.

Available agents Several compounds have been used for the management of myocardial infarction, of which three are readily available in the UK (Table 5.1):

● *Streptokinase*
Streptokinase—a product of *Streptococcus pyogenes* cultures—was the first thrombolytic agent to be studied. It forms a complex with plasminogen, and this combination converts further plasminogen molecules into their active form, plasmin. Being a foreign protein, streptokinase may occasionally

Table 5.1 ● Commonly used thrombolytic agents

Agent	Half-life (min)	Advantages	Disadvantages	Dose
Streptokinase	23	Inexpensive; widely used; chemically stable	Non-selective antigenic; less effective on old thrombus; requires infusion	1.5M units infused over 60 minutes
Anistreplase	90	Effective; easy administration as bolus; prolonged action	Relatively expensive; antigenic hypotension possible with rapid injection	30 mg as a bolus over 5 minutes
Alteplase (rt-PA)	5	Effective; relatively selective; non-antigenic	Requires infusion; expensive; short half-life	100mg given as; 10 mg bolus,then 50 mg infusion over 1st hour, then 40 mg infusion over next 2 hours

cause antigenic reactions; and antibodies preventing its therapeutic effect may limit the second use of this drug within a
time-window of 5 days to at least 12 months after the initial
dose.

- *Anistreplase*

Anistreplase was engineered as a complex molecule, containing streptokinase, plasminogen, and an 'anisoyl' group that
renders the complex inactive until *in vivo* hydrolysis takes
place. Two benefits accrue from this unusual structure: the
effect of the compound is sustained after a single bolus injection; and it has a relatively high affinity for fibrin-bound plasminogen.

- *t-PA*

Tissue plasminogen activator (t-PA) is a naturally occurring
protein made in tiny quantities by many tissues. It has a high
affinity for plasminogen in the vicinity of a fibrin clot, with
much less effect on circulating plasminogen. Most t-PA available for therapeutic use is manufactured by recombinant gene
technology based on human cell cultures. The commercially
available product is thus known as rt-PA—or 'alteplase'. Its
close similarity to an endogenous protein ensures a very low
level of antigenicity; but it suffers the disadvantage of a very
short half-life.

Other agents Urokinase and pro-urokinase (or single-chain
urokinase) also occur naturally, and were first identified in
human urine. They are non-antigenic, but produce a similar
effect on plasminogen and circulating fibrinogen as streptokinase. Neither is licensed in the United Kingdom for routine
use in acute myocardial infarction.

Other experimental agents are under development to
improve efficacy, clot selectivity, and duration of action,
while maintaining a minimum of antigenic effect. Consideration is also being given to combining established agents as a
single therapeutic intervention.

To hasten the effect of thrombolytic therapy, a variety of
dosing schedules are being explored using established or
novel compounds. Accelerated or 'front-loaded' regimens of
rt-PA have received particular attention. The administration of
rt-PA by either a single or double bolus technique undoubtedly improves early coronary patency—but the translation of

these experimental results into routine clinical practice awaits the results of further clinical trials.

Beneficial effects Thrombolytic agents, given by intracoronary or intravenous routes, cause lysis of recently formed coronary thrombus. Reperfusion rates (as a percentage of occluded arteries made patent by the drug) range between 33 per cent and 84 per cent. This variation reflects the use of different agents, varying routes of administration, and the different times chosen for coronary angiography before and after treatment. Quoted reperfusion rates should be seen as only one of several indicators of effective thrombolytic action.

Improved myocardial perfusion may not depend solely on restoring coronary patency. Prevention of clot extension, a systemic anticoagulant effect, a reduction in blood viscosity, and improved collateral flow may all enable 'rescue' reperfusion of the infarcting area. Indeed, the benefit of thrombolytic agents given late after the onset of major symptoms may depend more on these factors than on a primary effect on intraluminal clot.

A beneficial effect of thrombolytic agents on left ventricular function, enzyme release, and the electrocardiogram may seem predictable from their action on coronary flow. Yet these 'surrogate markers' of benefit have been surprisingly difficult to demonstrate. This may be explained in part by the techniques used for their assessment, and in part by the phenomenon of myocardial 'stunning', where the electrical and mechanical effects of infarction remain for days or weeks, but eventually regress completely.

In contrast, the major action of thrombolytic agents in reducing the mortality of myocardial infarction is not in doubt. Table 5.2, from the data of the Fibrinolytic Therapy Trialists' (FTT) Collaborative Group, shows the combined results of nine randomized controlled trials of thrombolytic therapy each entering more than 1000 patients. The trials included were GISSI-1, ISAM, AIMS, ISIS-2, ASSET, USIM, ISIS-3, EMERAS, and LATE and presented a total for study of 58 600 patients. Although—surprisingly—the mortality on days 0–1 of the attack was higher in the treated group than in the controls, the survival advantage during days 2–35 strongly outweighed this early effect; the final proportional reduction in mortality at 35 days due to thrombolysis was 18 per cent.

78 • Management of acute mycocardial infarction

Table 5.2 • Mortality reduction in acute myocardial infarction by the use of thrombolytic therapy. Data from an overview by the Fibrinolytic Therapy Trialists' (FTT) Collaborative Group of 9 randomized controlled trials each entering over 1000 patients (CI, 95 per cent confidence interval)

Day of death	No. of deaths		Percentage reduction in mortality (CI)	Benefit per 1000 patients (CI)
	Thrombolysis	Control		
0	695	554	−26(−38 to −13)	−5 (−7 to −2)
1	475	549	13 (2–25)	3 (0–5)
2–7	847	1100	23 (16–31)	9 (6–12)
8–35	803	1154	32 (24–39)	13 (10–16)
0–35	2820 (9.6%)	3357 (11.5%)	18 (13–23)	18 (13–23)

A word of caution. 'Percentage reduction in mortality' tells us little about the absolute number of lives saved by thrombolytic therapy. Mortality would be reduced by 25 per cent if 40 patients in a placebo group died but only 30 in a treated group—10 people saved; but a similar proportional reduction in mortality would also occur if placebo-group and treatment-group deaths were only 8 and 6, respectively—a saving of 2 patients overall. In the major trials of thrombolytic agents, placebo mortality is reported as 5.7–13.0 per cent. Reducing mortality by even 50 per cent means a saving, at best, of no more than 7 lives per 100 people treated. Enthusiasm for the early use of thrombolytic agents in acute myocardial infarction should not be dulled by this analysis; but these figures help to put the matter in a correct perspective.

Adverse effects The major adverse effect of thrombolytic therapy is predictable: haemorrhage, overt or concealed. Superficial bruising and minor bleeding around venepuncture sites are common evidence of thrombolytic effect. Minor soft tissue trauma in the few days prior to infarction can predispose to a surprising degree of secondary haemorrhage. (A head injury with bruising prior to admission is a relative contraindication to therapy.)

Major bleeding complications—sufficient to warrant transfusion or to prolong hospital stay—occur in about 5 per cent of patients. Bleeding is chiefly from the gastrointestinal tract, but may also result in haematuria, intramuscular or retroperitoneal haematomata, or pulmonary haemorrhage with haemoptysis. Arterial, and to a smaller extent, venous cannulation can result in extensive bruising, and needs to be approached with caution. For this reason it is best to avoid subclavian venepuncture while a patient is receiving thrombolytic therapy, and to exercise considerable care if approaching central venous cannulation by any other route.

Intracerebral haemorrhage occurs in up to 1 per cent of patients. It is often associated with abrupt headache, drowsiness, and focal neurological signs. In a few cases it is self-limiting and recovers completely; more often a permanent neurological deficit occurs, or the event proves fatal.

If a severe bleeding complication occurs, reversal of the clotting defect may be indicated by the use of tranexamic acid in a dose of 1 g by slow intravenous injection. This can be repeated after two hours if necessary. Fresh frozen plasma may also be indicated to correct the coagulation defect, and blood transfusion may also be required if the haemorrhage is severe.

The non-haemorrhagic complications of thrombolytic therapy are usually minor (see Box 5.1). Allergic reactions to streptokinase-containing agents are uncommon, and prophylactic steroid or antihistamine therapy is unnecessary. For the rare (<1 per cent) cases of anaphylaxis, conventional treatment with adrenaline and hydrocortisone is recommended.

Box 5.1 • Non-haemorrhagic complications of thrombolytic agents

- Allergy: skin rashes, vasculitis
- Anaphylaxis
- Reperfusion arrhythmias
- Purpura
- Peripheral emboli

Note:
The overall incidence of side-effects is low.
Reperfusion arrhythmias are common, but are almost always benign, and often indicate a beneficial action of the drug.

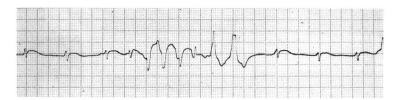

Fig. 5.8 ● Reperfusion arrhythmias following thrombolytic therapy.

Reperfusion arrhythmias are common (see Fig. 5.8), and can be a welcome indication of clot lysis. The overall incidence of life-threatening arrhythmias is reduced by thrombolysis; but those that do occur develop earlier in patients receiving active therapy than in controls. Reperfusion bradycardias (from reopening the right coronary artery) are usually transient and self-limiting, however, if prolonged they may warrant intravenous atropine. Heart block is not an absolute contraindication to thrombolysis; but careful thought needs to be given to the possible need, timing, and technique for temporary transvenous pacing.

Patient selection The selection of patients for thrombolysis rests on identifying those likely to be suffering from actual or imminent myocardial infarction due to coronary thrombosis, while noting any coexisting conditions that would increase the risk of therapy to unacceptable levels. No rigid criteria exist for patient selection, and no uniform policy has been adopted in the major mortality trials. A variation in approach will therefore be evident in clinical practice—but selection criteria will encompass age, the duration of pain, ECG abnormalities, and the presence of absolute or relative contraindications.

Typical cardiac pain is usually a prerequisite for thrombolytic therapy, but the time of onset of major symptoms can be difficult to determine, particularly if the course of the illness is stuttering. The symptom duration after which thrombolytic therapy is still judged worthwhile is more contentious. The marked value of early therapy is undoubted; but mortality studies have shown benefit with delays of up to 24 hours (ISIS-2). More recent trials suggest a practical cut-off for benefit of 12 hours.

The need for a characteristic ECG tracing is also contentious. An unequivocal infarct pattern (Fig. 5.3) poses no problem—and it identifies the patients most likely to gain from thrombolysis. Hyperacute changes (Fig. 5.4) also strongly indicate the use of thrombolytic therapy, but they may be more difficult to diagnose. In the face of a characteristic history, left-bundle branch-block should be taken as sufficient indication for thrombolysis, even without the additional ST segment elevation occasionally seen with this pattern (Fig. 5.6). Patients with ST segment depression alone (i.e. without ST elevation in any lead) seem not to benefit from thrombolytic therapy. However, although at least one major positive trial (ISIS-2) required no ECG criteria for admission, it seems wise to seek at least some electrocardiographic pointer to acute myocardial ischaemia.

An age-restriction was common during the early studies of thrombolytic therapy: but later work indicates increased benefit for the older patient. Age alone is no reason to withhold thrombolysis.

Box 5.2 ● Suggested indications for thrombolytic therapy

Definite
- Typical cardiac pain lasting more than 20 minutes
- Onset of major symptoms within 12 hours
- Characteristic ECG changes showing ST segment elevation:
    >2 mm in two contiguous precordial leads (not (V1)
    >1 mm in two limb leads representing the same wall of the ventricle
- Either gender
- Any age
- Any infarct site

Probable
- Typical symptoms with abnormal (preferably unstable) but not characteristic ECG
- Symptom duration 12–24 hours, with continuing pain and characteristic ECG

Box 5.2 summarizes the indications for the use of thrombolytic therapy, but local policies may differ and should always be consulted in practice.

Exclusion criteria (Box 5.3) are based primarily on identifying patients likely to suffer dangerous haemorrhage. Absolute contraindications are suspected aortic dissection and active bleeding. Recent major surgery and recent serious head-injury will also preclude the use of thrombolytic therapy in all but exceptional cases. The other conditions listed are relative, and need to be judged against the perceived benefit of thrombolysis in any individual patient. Diabetic retinopathy has also been listed, but in practice has proved to pose no real concern.

The safety of thrombolysis after CPR seems likely to depend on the duration of the resuscitation attempt. Successful resuscitation during the phase of 'three-quick-shocks-in-a-row' (pp. 20–1) should not preclude thrombolytic therapy. But prolonged attempts, for longer than 10 minutes, where continuing chest compression, intubation, and central venous cannulation have been necessary, are a contraindication. The grey area

---

Box 5.3 ● Contraindications to thrombolytic therapy

Absolute

- Suspected aortic dissection
- Active bleeding
- Use of anticoagulants/known bleeding diathesis
- Previous allergic reaction (streptokinase, anistreplase)
- Recent surgery or major trauma
- Recent head injury or cerebrovascular accident, even with complete recovery
- History of cerebrovascular accident with residual disability
- Abdominal aneurysm
- Prolonged cardiopulmonary resuscitation
- Possible pregnancy
- Systolic blood pressure > 180 mmHg
- Proliferative or haemorrhagic diabetic retinopathy

Relative

between 5 and 10 minutes offers a relative contraindication, in which the balance between benefit and haemorrhagic risk needs careful thought.

Practicalities of treatment: reducing delay and choice of agent Benefits from the use of thrombolytic therapy reduce with time. Delays are introduced progressively by the patient or relative, by pre-hospital evaluation and transport, and by the response of the receiving hospital. Unfortunately, initial patient delay seems difficult to influence even by widespread programmes of public instruction. Improvements in the response of general practitioners or the ambulance service through education and organizational change are easier to obtain.

The use of thrombolytic agents *before* hospital admission to reduce delay to therapy remains under debate. Pre-hospital administration undoubtedly shortens the delay to treatment, but the time gained varies substantially according to local geography, the nature of the first response system and the in-hospital delay at the receiving unit. (A long in-hospital delay will enhance the apparent advantages of pre-hospital care). Reported trials of pre-hospital thrombolysis show a range of times saved from about 30 minutes to more than 2 hours. Delays are shortened less in restricted, urban communities than in rural areas remote from hospital.

The largest trial to address the benefit of pre-hospital care has been the European Myocardial Infarction Project. Based on physician-manned mobile coronary care units, a total of 5469 patients from 16 countries were entered into a double-blind study of pre-hospital versus in-hospital administration of anistreplase for a clear presentation of acute myocardial infarction within 6 hours of the onset of symptoms. The time saved by pre-hospital treatment was a median of 55 minutes. The all-cause EMiP mortality at 30 days (the primary end-point of the trial) was reduced in the pre-hospital group by 13 per cent, but this figure did not reach statistical significance. Deaths from cardiac causes, however, were significantly less frequent in the pre-hospital group than in those treated after hospital arrival (8.3 vs. 5.8 per cent—a 16 per cent reduction).

The Grampian Region Early Anistreplase Trial (GREAT) explored the value of prehospital thrombolysis given by GPs in a rural area of Scotland. Although survival was not a primary end-point, the reduction in delay to thrombolytic therapy by 130 minutes through administration by GPs was associated with a 49 per cent reduction in mortality at 3 months as well as a demonstrable improvement in left ventricular function. Survival benefit was maintained at 1 year.

The message from these and other trials appears to be that the greatest clinical benefit occurs where the time to thrombolytic therapy can be reduced to less than 2 hours after the onset of symptoms. If this cannot be achieved (chiefly because of the patient's delay) outcome will be improved if an absolute reduction in delay to thrombolysis can be made of at least 60 and preferably 90 minutes through pre-hospital administration.

Several concerns remain about the use of pre-hospital thrombolysis in routine care: making an accurate diagnosis for patient selection, the possibility of serious adverse effects, the practicalities of administration, and the cost-effectiveness of implementing schemes for such 'advanced' pre-hospital care. However, trials to date have been reassuring on these points and many practitioners judge that thrombolysis at home is appropriate where patients are clearly eligible from the history and ECG, and where a substantial reduction in delay to treatment can be achieved, particularly within the first few hours of the attack. To adopt pre-hospital thrombolysis as routine, however, requires a more convenient thrombolytic agent, clear guidelines, adequate training, and close collaboration between all of the caring agencies involved.

An energetic commitment to early therapy and careful attention to practice are necessary to minimize the in-hospital delay to administering thrombolysis. Providing rapid patient assessment (triage) and giving thrombolytic therapy in the A&E Department are mandatory if the full benefits of thrombolysis are to be realized. Fortunately, the patients who stand to gain most will be the easiest to identify from their symptoms and characteristic ECG changes. Continuing audit of the delay time to therapy is also helpful in maintaining a pattern of rapid response.

The choice of thrombolytic agent may be determined by cost, local policy, participation in ongoing trials, and a history of previous use. Table 5.1 (p. 75) indicates the relative advantages and disadvantages of the currently available agents, together with recommended dose schedules.

Comparative efficacy has been studied recently in two important trials—GISSI-2 and ISIS-3. In GISSI-2, no important difference was found between the use of rt-PA and streptokinase, although some commentators feel that the results of this trial were weakened by a lack of concomitant heparin therapy. ISIS-3 similarly showed no difference in short-term mortality between patients treated with streptokinase, anistreplase, and rt-PA.

To address concerns that neither GISSI-2 nor ISIS-3 had used rt-PA in an optimal fashion (including the provision of an 'accelerated' dose schedule and early intravenous heparin), the GUSTO trial was conducted in just over 41 000 patients to compare four different thrombolytic regimens. These, with their case fatality rates, were:

Streptokinase plus SC heparin	7.2%
Streptokinase plus IV heparin	7.4%
Accelerated rt PA plus IV heparin	6.3%
Combined streptokinase and rt-PA	7.2%

The trial thus showed a 14 per cent reduction in 30-day mortality for the accelerated rt-PA regimen compared with the two streptokinase-only groups. This was at the expense, however, of a slight but significant increase in haemorrhagic stroke (0.72 vs. 0.54 per cent). Patients with anterior infarction appeared to benefit more than those with inferior infarction. In an angiographic sub-study of 2431 patients, patency of the infarct-related artery at 90 minutes was greater for the accelerated rt-PA regimen—although at 180 minutes appearances were similar between the different groups. Mortality improvement, as well as a lower incidence of arrhythmia, congestive heart failure, and shock was associated with the early re-opening of the culprit artery.

Although many practitioners acknowledge the superiority of an accelerated rt-PA-plus-heparin regimen it seems likely that on a cost–benefit basis streptokinase will retain its role in the UK as the first-line thrombolytic agent. Anistreplase may be helpful where administration by a single bolus is favoured, particularly in pre-hospital care; rt-PA will be useful for patients who have already received streptokinase or who have a strong history of allergy.

Thrombolytic therapy is often followed by the administration of heparin, though schedules for the timing and dose of this agent will vary from unit to unit.

Heparin

Seven per cent of patients hospitalized with chest pain from any cause develop subclinical peripheral venous thrombosis. The predisposition to deep vein thrombosis (DVT) rises steeply (to 17–38 per cent) if myocardial infarction is present, particularly if it is complicated by pericarditis, severe left ventricular failure, or cardiogenic shock. Heparin is useful for prophylaxis against venous thrombosis, and its routine use has virtually eliminated the fatalities that once occurred through massive pulmonary embolism.

In the arterial circulation heparin has two potential sites of beneficial effect: in the coronary artery, to limit the extension of intraluminal thrombosis; and in the left ventricle, to prevent mural thrombosis and consequent arterial embolism. With the advent of thrombolytic therapy heparin may have a new adjunctive role in maintaining coronary patency after clot lysis, although the likely importance of this role is currently debated.

For patients not receiving thrombolytic drugs a suitable schedule for heparin therapy is 40 000 units intravenously per day for 48 hours, starting as early in the admission as possible, and then 35 000 units per day until the patient is mobile. If mobility is delayed, maintenance heparin therapy by the subcutaneous route will be appropriate. Doses are reduced in the face of known peptic ulceration or any other increased risk of bleeding, or if the infarct is complicated by pericarditis.

Thrombolytic therapy reduces the requirement for heparin. A suggested regimen is to give 12 500 units subcutaneously twice a day, beginning 12 hours after thrombolysis, and continue this until the patient is mobile.

The use of heparin—even as a sole anticoagulant—is not without potential side-effects (Box 5.4), for which regular clinical review should be made. These adverse effects are particularly likely in a patient who has also received thrombolytic therapy.

Box 5.4 ● Adverse effect of heparin

● Haematomata
● Severe pain in sciatic or femoral nerve distribution
● Allergy
● Thrombocytopenia
● Haematuria
● Falling haemoglobin
● Retroperitoneal haemorrhage
● Unexplained peripheral vascular thrombosis

Anti-arrhythmic therapy

As will be outlined in Chapter 8 (p. 149), routine anti-arrhythmic therapy is no longer indicated in the management of acute myocardial infarction. A combination of several 'high-grade' ventricular arrhythmias or brief episodes of ventricular tachycardia in the first 24 hours warrants suppression with lignocaine, provided that the haemodynamic status permits. Aggressive arrhythmias require management as outlined in Chapter 7 (p. 119), with a preference for beta-blockers for important tachycardias related to re-infarction or ongoing ischaemia.

Bradycardia or block may require treatment with atropine or pacing, as is suggested in Box 5.5.

Beta blockers

In acute myocardial infarction beta blockers have three distinct areas of activity (see Box 5.6). Acutely, beta blockers lower heart rate and blood pressure, reducing myocardial oxygen demand. They have been shown to reduce coronary pain, lower ST elevation, and improve early mortality by substantially reducing the incidence of myocardial rupture. Trends showing a beneficial effect on re-infarction, cardiac arrest (in ventricular fibrillation), and ultimate infarct size have also been shown as a result of early beta blockade. But they should not be given to patients whose heart rate or blood pressure are depressed. The heart rate should be greater than 70/min and the systolic blood pressure greater than 100 mmHg, with a figure for (heart rate × systolic pressure) of greater than 10 000.

Box 5.5 • Treatment of bradycardias and block complicating acute myocardial infarction

Condition	Treatment
Rate <40/min	Atropine, pacing if ineffective
Poor haemodynamic state	
Pauses >3 seconds	
Bradycardia complicated by ventricular arrhythmias	Pacing
If subsidiary pacemaker has wide QRS, especially with RBBB pattern	Pacing

Note: AV block is considerably more worrying in anterior myocardial infarction than in an inferior infarct.

Box 5.6 •Uses of beta blockers in acute myocardial infarction

• In the first few hours of the attack as routine prophylaxis to limit mortality or myocardial damage;
• As treatment for recurrent cardiac pain or arrhythmias; and
• When the acute phase has passed, for the long-term reduction of mortality and re-infarction.

One suggested regimen is atenolol 5 mg intravenously over 5 minutes, repeated 15 minutes later in the absence of any adverse effects. At the same time commence oral therapy 50 mg twice daily for a total of 4 doses—or until a decision is made about the need for beta blockers for complications or as long-term secondary prevention.

Because of the negative effect of beta blockers on heart rate and contractility, and because of their potential non-cardiac side-effects, they cannot be used universally (see Box 5.7). Their use for the management of recurrent ischaemic chest pain following infarction is well established, and will usually

---

Box 5.7 • Contraindications to beta blockade early in acute myocardial infarction

- Heart rate: < 70 beats per minute
- Systolic blood pressure: <100 mmHg
- A rate–pressure product (heart rate × systolic blood pressure) <10 000
- Alveolar or interstitial oedema
- Known predisposition to bronchospasm
- Marked peripheral vascular disease
- Concurrent use of calcium-channel blockers, particularly verapamil

---

be associated with the concurrent use of nitrates, heparin, and aspirin. During the early stages of therapy attention should be paid to the possibility of worsening heart failure, and the need for more aggressive intervention if continuing ischaemia occurs in spite of maximum medical treatment.

Chronic beta blockade started early in the convalescent phase improves long-term outcome, particularly for those at high risk. These include patients with recurrent angina, late ventricular arrhythmias, poor left ventricular function, hypertension, or adverse findings on an exercise electrocardiogram. Patients with none of these risk factors have an extremely favourable one-year mortality; the use of routine long-term beta blockade (with its attendant side-effects) in this group is unwarranted.

Substantial evidence now exists that angiotensin-converting enzyme (ACE) inhibitors improve survival from myocardial infarction particularly when complicated by left ventricular failure (LVF). Data from many trials (SAVE, AIRE, TRACE, GISSI-3, ISIS-4, SMILE) demonstrate a proportional reduction in mortality of 6–27 per cent in patients treated with ACE inhibitors from within 24 hours to 11 days after their attack. Besides improving left ventricular remodelling, ACE inhibitors have an anti-ischaemic effect and afford long-term cardiac and vascular protection.

Debate continues over the best timing and necessary evidence to begin therapy, and about the most appropriate agent

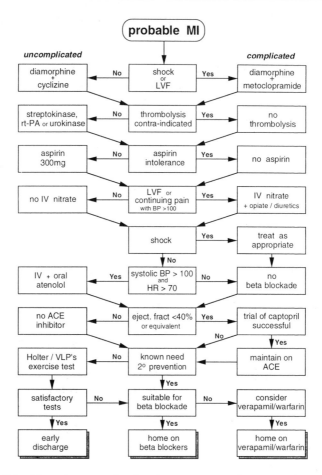

Fig. 5.9 • Flowchart—a plan for the treatment of suspected acute myocardial infarction.

to use. Introducing ACE inhibitors immediately on presentation of the infarct appears, on balance, to have an adverse effect. Many practitioners now consider day 2 (often within 24 hours), when haemodynamic stability has been achieved, to be optimum. Although the patients who benefit most are those with clinical, radiographic, or other investigational evidence of left ventricular failure, there is a growing tendency (in keeping with trial evidence) to introduce ACE inhibitors initially to a wider group of patients (say, all cases of anterior infarction) or even to *every* patient, at least until they can be shown to be at low risk.

In the absence of formal comparative trials, no particular agent appears substantially better than another: for the moment, the benefits of ACE inhibitors after myocardial infarction are judged to be a class effect. Whatever agent is used careful initial dosing is advised to avoid early, precipitous hypotension. In contrast, maintenance doses should be increased to as close to those used in published trials as possible, in order to secure the reported benefits in mortality.

Table 5.3 ● Common complications of acute myocardial infarction and the main therapeutic approaches to their management

Condition	Treatment
Left ventricular failure	Opoids, diuretics, nitrates, digoxin, inotropes, low-dose dopamine
Cardiogenic shock	Digoxin, low-dose dopamine, inotropes (e.g. dobutamine)
Heart block	Atropine, pacing
Ventricular tachycardia	Magnesium, lignocaine, procainamide, amiodarone
Pericarditis	Indomethacin
Recurrent cardiac pain	Nitrates, beta blockers, angiography
Hypertension	Beta blockers, nitrates, labetolol, nitroprusside
DVT, pulmonary embolism, arterial emboli	Heparin, later warfarin
Papillary muscle dysfunction	As for LVF, ?angiography if severe
Ventricular septal defect	As for shock, ?early angiography
Re-infarction	As for first episode; *consider* further thrombolysis

Treatment of complications

A detailed discussion of the complications of acute myocardial infarction and their treatment is inappropriate in a book predominantly about resuscitation. But Table 5.3 lists common complications, and the main therapeutic options for their management. Acute left ventricular failure is an emergency that should be treated early and aggressively, using oxygen with intravenous opioids, anti-emetics, nitrates, and diuretics. Consider early treatment with digoxin even for patients in sinus rhythm. The use of low-dose dopamine and intravenous inotropes may be necessary for the seriously ill patient, and should be used early where prior treatment with oral beta blockers has caused myocardial suppression.

Further reading

1. ACC/AHA Task Force (1990). Guidelines for the early management of patients with acute myocardial infarction. *Journal of the American College of Cardiology*, **16**, 249–92.
2. AIMS Trial Study Group (1988). Effect of intravenous anistreplase on mortality after acute myocardial infarction preliminary report of a placebo-controlled clinical trial. *Lancet*, **i**, 545–9.
3. Anderson, J. L. (ed.) (1989). Early intervention in the treatment of acute myocardial infarction—clinical profile of Eminase (APSAC). *American Journal of Cardiology*, **64** (Suppl.), 1–42A.
4. Braunwald, E. (1990). Optimising thrombolytic therapy of acute myocardial infarction. *Circulation*, **82**, 1510–13.
5. Braunwald, E. and Julian, D. (ed.) (1992). *Management of acute myocardial infarction*. Saunders, London.
6. Cleland, J. G. F. (1995). ACE inhibitors for myocardial infarction: how should they be used? *European Heart Journal*, **16**, 153–9.
7. de Bono, D. (1990). *Practical coronary thrombolysis*. Blackwell, Oxford.
8. Davies, M. J. and Thomas, A. C. (1985). Plaque fissuring—the cause of acute myocardial infarction, sudden ischaemic death, and crescendo angina. *British Heart Journal*, **53**, 363–73.
9. European Myocardial Infarction Group (1993). Prehospital thrombolitic therapy in patients with suspected acute myocardial infarction. *New England Journal of Medicine*, **329**, 383–85.

10. Fibrinolytic Therapy Trialists' (FIT) Collaborative Group (1994). Indications for fibrinolytic therapy in suspected acute myocardial infarction: collaborative overview of early mortality and major morbidity results from all randomised trials of more than 1000 patients. *Lancet*, **343**, 311–22.
11. Francis, G. S. (ed.) (1995). The role of ACE inhibitors in myocardial infarction—potential mechanisms and clinical implications. *European Heart Journal*, **16**(suppl. K), 1–54.
12. Grampion Region Early Anistreplase Trial Group (1992). Feasibility, safety, and efficacy of domiciliary thrombolysis by general practitioners: Grampion Region Early Anistreplase Trial. *British Medical Journal*, **305,** 548–53.
13. GUSTO Investigators (1993). An international randomised trial comparing four thrombolytic strategies for acute myocardial infarction. *New England Journal of Medicine*, **329**, 673–82.
14. Hands, M. E., Cook, E. F., Stone, P. H., Muller, J. E., Hartwell, T., Sobel, B. E., *et al.* (1988). Electrocardiographic diagnosis of myocardial infarction in the presence of complete left bundle branch block. *American Heart Journal*, **61**, 9–13.
16. ISIS-1 (First International Study of Infarct Survival). Collaborative Group (1986). Randomised trial of intravenous atenolol among 16 027 cases of suspected acute myocardial infarction: ISIS-1. *Lancet*, **ii**, 57–66.
17. ISIS-1 (First International Study of Infarct Survival) Collaborative Group. (1988). Mechanisms for the early mortality reduction produced by beta-blockade started early in acute myocardial infarction: ISIS-1. *Lancet*, **i**, 921–3.
18. ISIS-2 (Second International Study of Infarct Survival) Collaborative Group. (1988). Randomised trial of intravenous streptokinase, oral aspirin, both or neither among 17 187 cases of suspected acute myocardial infarction: ISIS-2. *Lancet*, **i**, 349–60.
19. ISIS-3 (Third International Study of Infarct Survival) Collaborative Group. (1993). ISIS-3: a randomised comparison of streptokinase vs. tissue plasminogen activator vs. anistreplase and of aspirin plus heparin vs. aspirin alone among 41 299 cases of suspected acute myocardial infarction. *Lancet*, **339**, 753–70.
20. Lee, H. S., Cross, S. J., Garthwait, P., *et al.* (1994). Comparison of the value of a novel rapid measurement of myoglobin, creatine kinase, and creatine kinase-MB with the electrocardiogram for the diagnosis of acute myocardial infarction. *British Heart Journal*, **71**, 311–15.
21. MacCallum, A. G., Stafford, P. J., Jones, C., Vincent, R., Perez-Avila, C., and Chamberlain, D. A. (1990). Reduction in hospital

time to thrombolytic therapy by audit of policy guidelines. *European Heart Journal*, **11**, 48–52.

22. Massel, D., Gill, J. B. and Cairns, J. A. (1990). Management of the patient following coronary thrombolysis. *Annals of Cardiology*, **13**, 591–609.

23. Norwegian Multicenter Study Group (1982). Timolol-induced reduction in mortality and reinfarction in patients surviving acute myocardial infarction. *New England Journal of Medicine*, **304**, 891–7.

24. Pepise, C. J. (1989). New concepts in the pathophysiology of AMI. *American Journal of Cardiology*, **64**, 2–8B.

25. Purvis, J. A., McNeill, A. J., Siddiqui, R. A., *et al.* (1994). Efficacy of 100 mg of double-bolus alteplase in achieving complete perfusion in the treatment of acute myocardial infarction. *Journal of the American College of Cardiology*, **23**, 6–10.

26. Schweitzer, P. (1990). The electrocardiographic diagnosis of myocardial infarction in the thrombolytic era. *American Heart Journal*, **119**, 642–54.

27. Sleight, P. and Chamberlain, D. A. (ed.) (1990). *Thrombolysis: the dawn of a new era?* IBC Technical Services, London.

28. Weston, C. G. M., Penny, W. J. and Julian, D. G. (1994). Guidelines for the management of patients with myocardial infarction. *British Medical Journal*, **308**, 767–71.

29. White, P. W., Sadd, J. R., and Nense, R. E. (1979). Thrombotic complications of heparin therapy: including six cases of heparin-induced skin necrosis. *Annals of Surgery*, **190**, 595–608.

30. Wilcox, R. G., von der Lippe, G., Olsson, C. G., Jensen, G., Skene, A. M. and Hampton, J. R. (1988). Trial of tissue plasminogen activator for mortality reduction in acute myocardial infarction: Anglo-Scandinavian study of early thrombolysis (ASSET). *Lancet*, **ii**, 525–30.

31. Yusuf, S., Collins, R., MacMahon, S. and Peto, R. (1988). Effect of intravenous nitrates on mortality in acute myocardial infarction: an overview of the randomised trials. *Lancet*, **i**, 1088–92.

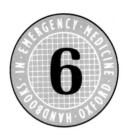

CHAPTER 6

Ventilation and intravenous cannulation

Key points in airway management and ventilation

1 A patent and secure airway is of paramount importance during cardiopulmonary resuscitation.

2 Mouth-to-mouth breathing provides adequate ventilation and requires no equipment.

3 Incorrect use of the oropharyngeal airway may further occlude the airway.

4 A two-person technique is preferred for effective bag-valve-facemask ventilation.

5 Always auscultate the chest to ensure effective ventilation of both lungs after endotracheal intubation.

6 Surgical cricothyroidotomy, although rarely indicated, is straightforward to perform and may be life-saving.

Key points in drug-delivery routes and intravenous cannulation

1 Central venous injection of drugs during cardiopulmonary resuscitation is the preferred route.

2 Peripheral circulation during external cardiac compression is sluggish, and therefore peripherally injected drugs are slow to reach their site of action.

3 There is little evidence that administration of drugs via the endotracheal route is effective during resuscitation of the cardiac-arrested human.

4 Intracardiac injections are not recommended.

Airway management and ventilation

Importance of adequate oxygenation and airway care

Adequate oxygenation of the patient during resuscitation is paramount. This requires the presence of four separate components:

1. an adequate upper airway;
2. an adequate lower airway;
3. adequate 'tidal' ventilation (to ensure carbon dioxide removal as well as oxygen provision); and
4. an increased delivered oxygen concentration (F_iO_2).

It is important to point out that the fully conscious non-arrested patient suffering an acute myocardial infarction or trauma also needs care of the airway and oxygen. All too often such patients, because they are breathing, are denied the opportunity of enhanced inspired oxygen concentrations—a deprivation which is likely to be to their detriment. The airway must be protected against inhalation of vomit.

There are a variety of methods of ventilating the cardiac-arrested patient, and the method used will depend on: the circumstances of the arrest; the skill levels available for airway control; and the availability of an appropriate form of airway for the individual patient.

Airway care can be conveniently divided into:

(1) basic airway care—with or without adjuncts; and
(2) advanced airway care.

Basic airway care

Expired air respiration (EAR).

Disadvantages of expired air respiration
Direct mouth-to-mouth breathing (Expired Air Respiration—EAR) is the commonest form of ventilation for a patient managed by a layperson out of hospital. This is an excellent and proven method of ventilation, but has certain disadvantages. First, the inspired oxygen concentration for the patient is usually no more than 16 per cent; and, secondly, particularly in the presence of vomit, the rescuer may find the method

extremely unpleasant. There is, however, no evidence of transmission of significant infection via this route. For example, there has been no proven case of transmission of the human immunodeficiency virus (HIV) as a result of mouth-to-mouth breathing.

Box 6.1 • Disadvantages of expired air respiration

- Low F_iO_2—16 per cent
- Unpleasant for rescuer

Technique of expired air respiration
The technique of EAR recommended by the Resuscitation Council (UK) is as follows:

1. With the patient lying supine, obvious obstructions, including broken or displaced dentures, should be removed from the mouth. Well-fitting dentures should normally be left in place, as they provide a better mouth-to-mouth seal.
2. The head should be gently tilted back and the mouth opened. While kneeling by the patient's head, the rescuer should, with one hand, pinch the nose, and, with the other, support the jaw. The rescuer should then take a breath and
3. . . . place his or her mouth completely over the patient's mouth, making a firm seal. The rescuer should then breathe into the patient.
4. Two slow, full breaths should be given, each sufficient to cause the chest to rise. Between inflations the chest should be allowed to fall while the rescuer turns his or her head to one side. (See Figs 6.1–6.3.)

If the chest does not rise with each breath then either the airway is obstructed or a satisfactory mouth-seal has not been achieved. The airway should be reassessed or the seal should be improved before continuing.

After these two breaths the cartid pulse should be checked. If the pulse is absent, chest compressions and EAR should be performed in a ratio of 15 compressions: 2 ventilations at a rate sufficient to provide 4 cycles per minute. If a pulse is pre-

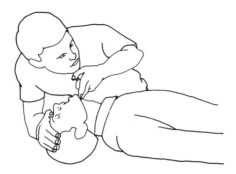

Fig. 6.1 ● Position of rescuer and victim just prior to commencement of expired air resuscitation (EAR).

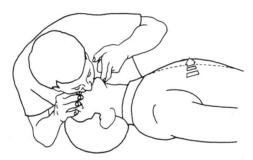

Fig. 6.2 ● Expired air resuscitation (EAR) being administered.

sent but the casualty is still not breathing, EAR should be continued at a rate of about 12 breaths per minute.

Airway care adjuncts

Guedel airway The airway of the self-ventilating, but unconscious, patient may be adequately maintained by using a Guedel airway. In the cardiac-arrested and apnoeic patient, however, it must be used in conjunction with a means of ventilating the patient.

The size of Guedel oropharyngeal airway necessary can be assessed by placing the airway against the patient's face. The

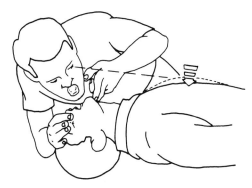

Fig. 6.3 • Rescuer observes victim's chest falling between each ventilation.

correct-sized airway will extend from the centre of the patient's mouth to the angle of the jaw.

After opening the patient's mouth the airway is inserted with its convex surface against the anterior part of the patient's tongue. As the airway is further advanced it is rotated through 180 degrees into its correct position. The lips and tongue must not be caught between the teeth and the Guedel airway.

It is important to select the correct size of Guedel airway—too long an airway may reach the epiglottis, push it posteriorly, and thus occlude the larynx. If the airway is inserted incorrectly, without rotation, it may push the tongue backwards, further occluding the airway.

Laerdal pocket mask The Laerdal pocket mask, Fig. 6.4, is a very useful piece of inexpensive equipment for the layperson as well as nursing, paramedical, and medical staff.

The mask is packaged in a collapsed state, in which it can easily be carried in a pocket or the glove-compartment of a car. It has a one-way valve and a securing elastic head-strap. The mask is placed in position and held securely with two hands, while the rescuer simultaneously produces jaw-thrust (Fig. 6.5). Ventilation can then be given effectively without direct mouth-to-mouth contact, thus avoiding the exhaled air being inhaled by the rescuer. In the presence of an oxygen

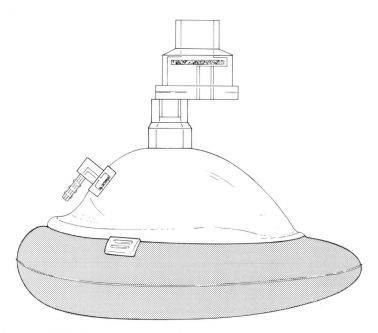

Fig. 6.4 ● The Laerdal pocket mask, with oxygen side port, assembled and ready for use.

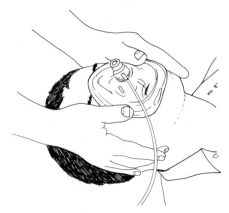

Fig. 6.5 ● The Laerdal pocket mask in use.

supply, supplementary oxygen can be provided, via an oxygen port, to enhance the inspired oxygen concentration administered to the patient. To improve the adequacy of ventilation still further this mask can be used in conjunction with a Guedel airway.

Bag-valve-mask technique In addition to the mouth-to-face-mask technique of ventilation, the bag-valve-mask technique can be used, and is preferentially to be employed in hospital. A Guedel airway should be inserted prior to its use. A two-person technique improves effectiveness substantially, with one operator holding the facemask in place and simultaneously producing jaw-thrust, while the other uses both hands to squeeze the bag. Supplemental oxygen can be delivered via an oxygen port in the ventilation bag. Pre-oxygenation, using the bag-valve-mask technique with a Guedel airway in place, should be performed before endotracheal intubation is attempted.

Advanced airway care

There are two methods of securing the airway during cardiopulmonary resuscitation. By far the more common of these is tracheal intubation; but very rarely cricothyroidotomy may be indicated. These will be discussed in turn.

Tracheal intubation Patients suffering a cardiopulmonary arrest out of hospital may have been intubated during resuscitation by ambulance personnel or pre-hospital-care doctors. Other patients may only have received basic airway care.

A patent and secure airway is of paramount importance during cardiopulmonary resuscitation.

Tracheal intubation technique Having checked the correct operation of the laryngoscope, and in particular that the light source is adequate and the bulb is not loose, the open laryngoscope is held in the left hand (Fig. 6.6).

A 7 or 8 mm internal diameter endotracheal tube should be selected for a woman, and an 8 or 9 mm internal diameter tube for a man.

The patient's head should be extended at the atlanto-occipital joint, and the neck should be flexed—the 'sniffing the morning air' position. This position may be facilitated by placing a small pillow under the patient's head.

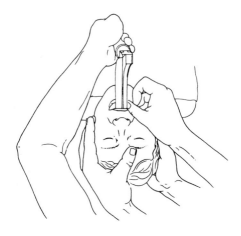

Fig. 6.6 ● Tracheal intubation technique—insertion of the laryngoscope.

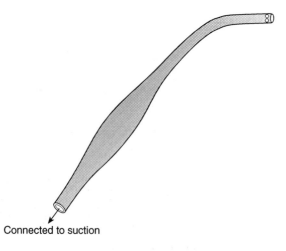

Connected to suction

Fig. 6.7 ● The Yankauer (rigid) suction catheter.

The upper airway should be cleared of any fluid or vomit using a rigid Yankauer sucker (Fig. 6.7). Suction can be provided by portable, battery-operated or manual devices in the pre-hospital phase or during transport within hospital. Mobile, mains-operated suction units are available for hospital use; or, alternatively, piped wall suction may be used.

The curved laryngoscope blade is inserted over the right-hand surface of the patient's tongue. This will gently move the tongue to the left. The laryngoscope is advanced over the anterior and then the posterior portion of the tongue until its tip reaches the vallecula (Fig. 6.8). The vallecula is sited at the junction between the base of the tongue and the epiglottis. The tongue and lower jaw are then lifted gently anteriorly. The epiglottis will move anteriorly to expose the vocal cords (Fig. 6.9). The endotracheal tube is inserted through the cords under direct vision. The cuff is inflated, and the tube is secured in place. Ventilation using a bag-valve device with supplemental oxygen can then proceed.

The correct positioning of the tube must be checked by auscultating both sides of the chest and the stomach. If the tube has been inserted too far, the right main bronchus may have been intubated, resulting in air entry into the right chest only. If this is the case the tube should be gently withdrawn, and the adequacy of ventilation rechecked.

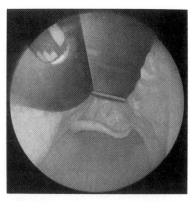

Fig. 6.8 • Tip of the laryngoscope blade in the vallecula, between the base of the tongue and the base of the epiglottis.

Occasionally, intubation by standard methods proves impossible, and other techniques such as the use of a malleable bougie may be considered (Fig. 6.10). This is passed under laryngoscopic direct vision between the vocal cords. The endotracheal tube is then 'rail-roaded' over the bougie.

Complications of tracheal intubation
1. Oesophageal intubation, which, if it occurs and is not recognized, will result in progressive hypoxia and death. The

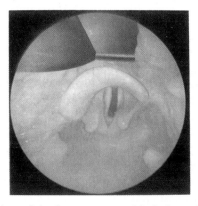

Fig. 6.9 ● Elevation of the laryngoscope blade in order to visualize clearly the vocal cords and the entrance to the larynx.

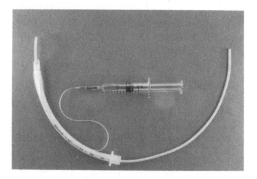

Fig. 6.10 ● Gum elastic bougie and endotracheal tube.

use of an end tidal carbon dioxide detection device will alert the clinician to inadvertent oesophageal intubation.

2. Intubation of one main bronchus, commonly the right.
3. Damage to structures, particularly the teeth, tongue, and upper larynx.
4. A poorly inflated endotracheal tube cuff, or leaking cuff, leading to inadequate ventilation. The airway is also not protected against aspiration.

The laryngeal mask airway was introduced into anaesthetic practice in 1988. It is now widely used in anaesthesia, both in the United Kingdom and abroad. It has not yet, however, achieved acceptance as a useful airway adjunct during cardiopulmonary resuscitation. This situation may change. The laryngeal mask must not, and cannot be seen as an alternative to tracheal intubation, as it cannot *protect* the airway against aspiration. It may well find a use as a more effective alternative to mask ventilation before a clinician capable of tracheal intubation arrives.

Training
Practical training is an essential prerequisite for successful airway care in the demanding circumstances of a cardiorespiratory arrest. This is particularly true of endotracheal intubation.

Training in endotracheal intubation should begin on mannequins and be followed, ideally, on anaesthetized patients under the direction of a skilled anaesthetist. This latter form of training is not available to all those who may suddenly be required to provide airway care in an emergency. The use of human cadavers, after an unsuccessful resuscitation attempt, for this purpose is controversial. Under controlled, dignified circumstances, however, and after explanation and discussion with all concerned, particularly the nursing staff, such training is invaluable—the benefit may be successful airway care in a subsequent patient.

Surgical cricothyroidotomy Very rarely, for instance when an inhaled foreign body impacts in the upper airway, tracheal intubation is not possible by the above methods. In these circumstances a surgical airway is required. The surgical cricothyroidotomy technique is simple to perform, and may be life-saving in these situations (Fig. 6.11).

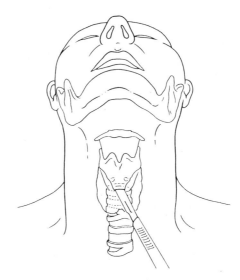

Fig. 6.11 ● Transverse incision for cricothyroidectomy, between the thyroid and cricoid cartilage, through the cricothyroid membrane.

In an increasingly litigious United Kingdom it may be insufficient to say that endotracheal intubation was unsuccessful, given that there is another easily available route for securing an airway. Individual Districts and their Resuscitation Committees must decide whether cricothyroidotomy should be advocated.

Surgical cricothyroidotomy technique Suction must be available during this procedure, to remove both blood from the incision and secretions released when the cricothyroid membrane is incised.

1. Surgically prepare the skin overlying the larynx.
2. Whilst stabilizing the larynx between the index finger and thumb of the left hand, palpate the cricothyroid membrane.
3. Incise the skin transversely over the cricothyroid membrane, and then carefully incise the membrane itself.
4. Enlarge the opening gently with a tracheal spreader, and insert a 5 or 6 mm internal diameter cuffed tracheostomy tube.

5. Inflate the balloon and secure the tube in place.
6. Ventilate the patient.

Drug-delivery routes and intravenous cannulation

The use of needles, particularly in the circumstances of management of cardiac arrest, raises the possibility of needle-stick injury. There are a variety of precautions that should be taken, especially in the A&E department:

1. Ensure that all A&E staff (doctors, nurses, medical students) are immunized against hepatitis B.
2. Each individual should dispose of his or her sharps immediately after use.
3. Resheathing of needles should, ideally, be avoided under all circumstances—if absolutely essential, place the unheld sheath on a work surface and direct the needle into it.

During the course of the management of a cardiac arrest drugs have been given via a variety of routes:

(1) via a central venous cannula;
(2) via a peripheral venous cannula;
(3) via an intravenous needle in children;
(4) via an intraosseus needle;
(5) in droplet form via an endotracheal tube; and
(6) directly into the heart via an intracardiac needle.

Patients suffering a cardiac arrest may have a peripheral cannula in place; if so, this should be used for drug administration until a central route has been established. This will depend on the skill levels available. However, ideally, the team should include a clinician capable of inserting a central venous cannula.

Intravenous cannulation:

Peripheral versus central intravenous drug administration

Although some animal studies suggest there is little difference in the effectiveness of central rather than peripheral intravenous injection routes, Kuhn showed a substantial delay in arrival of dye in the femoral artery following peripheral intravenous administration in cardiac-arrested humans. Dye injected centrally showed a high concentration in the femoral artery within 30 seconds. Peripherally injected dye was not present at the femoral artery at 90 seconds. Central venous injection of drugs during cardiopulmonary resuscitation is, therefore, the preferred route.

Types of intravenous cannulae The cannulae available for intravenous administration of drugs are:

1. Cannula over needle–(a) a combined cannula and needle inserted;
   –(b) needle withdrawn, leaving plastic cannula in vein.
2. *Hollow needle*—i.e. butterfly device, leaving needle in vein.
3. *Cannula through needle*–needle sited intravenously, and plastic cannula passed through the needle to be sited in the vein.
4. *Seldinger technique*–(a) Hollow needle sited intravenously;
   –(b) guide wire passed through needle into vein;
   –(c) needle withdrawn;
   –(d) plastic cannula inserted over guide wire into vein.

The cannula over the needle device is most commonly used during cardiopulmonary resuscitation. It is far quicker than the cannula through the needle or the Seldinger technique. Also, it does not suffer from the disadvantage of the hollow-needle device, which may well dislodge during vigorous resuscitation.

Although sterile precautions must be taken when siting intravenous cannulae, the circumstances of the cardiac arrest may render an absolutely aseptic technique difficult. Certainly, following a successful resuscitation, all intravenous cannulae should be resited in a sterile fashion.

Central venous cannulation

The internal jugular vein or the subclavian vein can be cannulated; but the internal jugular route is to be preferred, as cannulation of this vein does not interfere with continuing external cardiac massage. Whilst assessing the neck before cannulation, the external jugular vein may be noted to be distended. Cannulation of this vein may be possible, and less problematic than internal jugular vein cannulation. The onset of the action of drugs by the external jugular route, will be delayed compared to the internal jugular, but be quicker than a peripheral venous injection. The femoral vein may also be used but has no advantage over a peripheral vein, unless a long catheter is used to ensure rapid drug delivery.

Internal jugular vein cannulation (central approach) During cardiopulmonary resuscitation (CPR) the patient will necessarily be in the supine position. Reduced cardiac output resulting from the relative ineffectiveness of external cardiac compression compared with the patient's previous inherent cardiac output results in central venous engorgement and a raised central venous pressure. A head-down position is, therefore, neither necessary nor convenient.

The equipment needed is:

(1) 5¼″ cannula over needle (14G);
(2) 10 ml syringe;
(3) alcohol swabs for skin cleansing; and
(4) 500 ml 5 per cent glucose with giving set already run through.

Surface anatomy of the internal jugular vein The surface anatomy of the internal jugular vein is represented by a line drawn from the lobule of the ear to the medial end of the clavicle. During its course it lies directly underneath a depression formed between the sternal and clavicular heads of the sternocleidomastoid muscle in the lower part of the neck (Fig. 6.12).

Although there are three approaches to the internal jugular vein, namely the posterior, central, and anterior, the central approach is preferred, and will be described.

There are definite advantages in cannulating the right internal jugular vein because:

(1) the thoracic duct which runs on the left side of the neck is not endangered;
(2) the dome of the pleura, although still at risk of puncture, is not as high on the right as the left; and

(3) the drainage of the right internal jugular vein, eventually into the superior vena cava, follows a more direct course.

Once the necessary equipment has been collected internal jugular vein cannulation via the central approach can be attempted. Resuscitation should continue, defibrillation being the only procedure which will interrupt internal jugular vein cannulation.

Technique for cannulation of the internal jugular vein
1. Rotate the patient's head gently 30 degrees to the left.
2. Identify the triangle formed by the sternal head of sterno-cleidomastoid medially, the clavicular head laterally, and the medial portion of the clavicle inferiorly. If it cannot easily be seen the triangular depression can be palpated. Identify the *apex* of this triangle superiorly.
3. Clean the skin, and connect the 10 ml syringe to the cannula.
4. Puncture the skin at the apex of the triangle.

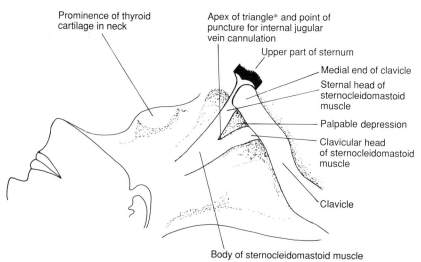

*Triangle formed by sternal head and clavicular head of sternocleidomastoid and the medial portion of the clavicle

Fig. 6.12 • Surface anatomy of the neck for internal jugular vein cannulation.

5. Expel the small skin-plug which may lodge in the needle tip with 1 ml of air.
6. With the needle-tip *just* subcutaneous, and the cannula at 30 degrees to the skin, advance the needle slowly towards the right nipple, keeping gentle suction on the syringe. The vein should be entered within 3 cm. Further advance will be hazardous, particularly to the dome of the right pleura.
7. On entering the vein a free flow, or 'flashback', of blood will appear in the syringe.
8. Advance the needle and cannula a few millimetres further.
9. Withdraw on the syringe again to confirm the needle cannula tip is still in the vein.
10. Without further advance at this stage, gently realign the cannula, pointing it towards the right sternoclavicular joint—the cannula will then be aligned with the vein.
11. Withdraw on the syringe, to again confirm continued presence in the vein.
12. Advance the cannula over the needle with an oscillating motion on the cannula hub. The cannula should advance easily over the needle. Resistance implies unsuccessful cannulation.
13. Once the cannula has been fully advanced ensure the giving set is ready to connect.
14. Remove the needle/syringe and quickly connect the giving set to the cannula.
15. Fully turn on the giving set.
16. Secure the cannula in place with a large transparent adhesive dressing.
17. Finally, to confirm central venous access, lower the bag of 5 per cent glucose to the floor, and, with the flow still turned on, blood will reverse down the giving set.
18. Return the 5 per cent glucose bag to the drip stand.
19. Drugs can now be given, via the giving-set hub and through the central venous cannula, virtually into the right atrium of the heart.

Subclavian vein cannulation The approach to the subclavian vein inhibits effective external cardiac compression. It is not, therefore, recommended, unless cannulation of the internal jugular vein has not been successful.

Similar equipment to that used for internal jugular vein cannulation may be used:

(1) 5¼″ cannula over needle (14G);
(2) 10 ml syringe;
(3) alcohol swabs for skin cleansing; and
(4) 500 ml of 5 per cent glucose connected to a giving set, run through and ready to connect.

Surface anatomy of the subclavian vein The surface anatomy of the subclavian vein can be represented by a broad line running behind the clavicle from a little inside its midpoint to the medial edge of the clavicular head of the sternocleidomastoid.

Technique for cannulation of the subclavian vein

1. The arrested patient will be in the supine position. Central venous engorgement will be present because of high venous pressure.
2. Having connected the cannula to the syringe, identify the junction between the middle and medial thirds of the clavicle.
3. Clean the skin area of the proposed cannulation site with alcohol swabs.
4. With the syringe and needle held in the frontal plane, introduce the needle approximately 1 cm below the junction of the middle and medial thirds of the clavicle. Expel the small skin-plug with 1 ml of air.
5. Apply gentle suction on the syringe.
6. Direct the needle medially and slightly cephalad (upwards) behind the clavicle, aiming towards a point just below a fingertip placed in the suprasternal notch.
7. Once the vein has been entered (confirmed by blood entering the syringe) advance the cannula over the needle.
8. Ensuring that the giving set is ready for connection, rapidly remove the needle and connect the giving set to the cannula.
9. Secure the cannula in place with a large transparent adhesive dressing.
10. With the tap turned on, lower the bag of 5 per cent glucose to the floor to ensure a ready flashback of blood into the giving set confirming satisfactory venous cannulation.
11. Replace the 5 per cent glucose bag on the drip stand.
12. Drugs can now be given centrally via the giving-set hub.

Box 6.2 • Complications of central venous cannulation

- Pneumothorax
- Haemopneumothorax
- Air embolus
- Damage to local structures
- Chylothorax

Pneumothorax caused during central line insertion will rapidly become a tension pneumothorax during positive pressure ventilation. *Haemopheumothorax* is a particular risk of central line placement via the subclavian route. *Air embolus* is a definite hazard for the non-cardiac-arrested patient unless a 15 degree head-down position is ensured. The arrested patient may remain horizontal as venous engorgement is assured because of high venous pressure secondary to a poor cardiac output during external chest compression.

As well as *local problems*, such as haemotoma formation, phlebitis, thrombosis, and cellulitis, *local structures*, such as the carotid artery during jugular vein cannulation, may be damaged. Finally, *chylothorax* may be caused by damage to the thoracic duct on the left side of the root of the neck.

Peripheral venous route

If a peripheral intravenous route is used for drug administration during cardiopulmonary resuscitation, remember that the peripheral circulation with external cardiac compression will be sluggish. Ninety to 120 seconds should be allowed for the drug to reach its site of action, during which time ventilation and external cardiac massage must continue. Further delay will occur unless the arm in which the cannula is inserted is elevated, and the drug is flushed into the circulation with 5 per cent glucose solution.

Intraosseus route

The intraosseus route (also described in Chapter 9) can be used in children less than 6 years of age. This route is increasing in popularity and is indicated in an emergency, such as cardiac arrest, when two attempts at venous cannulation have failed.

The technique is save, effective, and quick, but *sterile precautions* must be taken. Intraosseus access is gained as follows;

1. Identify the correct anatomical site. The preferred site is the anterior, subcutaneous part of the tibia, one fingerbreadth below the tibial tuberosity (a low femoral approach may be used in the trauma situation when there is an ipsilateral tibial fracture).
2. The chosen site is cleaned, and a small skin incision made to ease introduction of the intraosseus needle.
3. A 16G or 18G spinal needle, or a specially manufactured intraosseus needle, at least 1.5″ long is selected.
4 The needle is inserted anteriorly, at right angles to the tibia, with a gyratory motion, until a 'give' is felt on entering the bone marrow cavity.
5 The marrow cavity is aspirated with a 5 ml syringe in order to confirm entry.
6. Drugs (or crystalloids and blood products in trauma) can be given directly into the marrow cavity. They must be given, under pressure, from a syringe.

The intraosseus needle should be removed as soon as possible as the only significant complication is local cellulitis or, rarely, osteomyelitis.

Endotracheal route

In out-of-hospital cardiac arrest management it is often difficult to establish intravenous access. Endotracheal administration of lignocaine, adrenaline, and atropine in droplet form has therefore been advocated. Bray showed an encouraging response to intratracheal atropine in anaesthetized patients—the onset of tachycardia was quicker than with a peripheral intravenous infusion. However, in the cardiac-arrested human Quinton has shown no rise in arterial adrenaline levels following intratracheal injection, compared with a threefold rise following a peripheral intravenous injection. Intratracheal administration of drugs in the cardiac-arrested human is, therefore, at best inferior to peripheral intravenous infusion, and, at worst, ineffective.

Intracardiac injections

Transthoracic intracardiac injections have no place in modern cardiopulmonary resuscitation. In the past they have been advocated as a last resort. Sabin traced the intracardiac injection site or sites in 18 patients dying after unsuccessful cardiopulmonary resuscitation. Of the 46 injections carried out, only 18 punctured the left or right ventricle. Complications of the procedure include coronary artery laceration, pneumothorax, haemopericardium, haemothorax, and intramyocardial injection.

Although it is possible that Sabin's series may have preferentially selected unsuccessful attempts at intracardiac injection, given the potential complications and the relatively low success rate, intracardiac injection is not recommended.

Further reading

1. Barsan, W. G., Levy, R. C. and Weir, H. (1981). Lidocaine levels during CPR: differences after peripheral venous, central venous and intracardiac injections. *Annals of Emergency Medicine*, **10**, 73–8.
2. Barsan, W. G., Hedges, J. R., Nishijama, H., and Lukes, S. T. (1986). Differences in drug delivery with peripheral and central venous injections: normal perfusion. *American Journal of Emergency Medicine*, **4**, 1–3.
3. Bray, B. M., Jones, H. M. and Grundy, E. M. (1987). Tracheal versus intravenous atropine. *Anaesthesia*, **42**, 1188–90.
4. Kuhn, G. J., White, B. C., Swetnam, R. E., Mumey, J. F., Rydesky, M. F., Tintinally, J. E., *et al.* (1981). Peripheral vs. central circulation times during CPR. *Annals of Emergency Medicine*, **10**, 417–19.
5. *Lancet* (Editorial) (1988). Intratracheal drugs. *Lancet*, **i**, 743–4.
6. Quinton, D. N., O'Byrne, G., and Aitkenhead, A. R. (1987). Comparison of endotracheal and peripheral IV adrenaline in cardiac arrest. *Lancet*, **i**, 828–9.
7. Royal College of Physicians (1987). *Resuscitation from cardiopulmonary arrest. Training and organisation*. The Royal College of Physicians, London.
8. Sabin, H. I., Coghill, S. B., Khunti, K. and McNeil, G. O. (1983). Accuracy of intracardiac injections determined by a post-mortem study. *Lancet*, **ii**, 1054–5.
9. Skinner, D., Driscoll, P. and Earlam, R. (ed.) (1994). *ABC of major trauma*, (2nd edn). British Medical Journal, London.

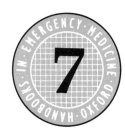

CHAPTER 7

Management of common arrhythmias associated with cardiac arrest

Key points in the management of arrhythmias

1 A clear trace showing distinct P waves and QRS complexes is mandatory for arrhythmia diagnosis.

2 A 12-lead ECG is essential for the management of tachycardias associated with a broad QRS complex.

3 The treatment for tachyarrhythmias associated with profound haemodynamic collapse is an urgent DC shock. The initial energy chosen, the use of synchronization, and the choice of any associated drug therapy depend on a correct interpretation of the presenting rhythm.

4 Where the mechanism of a broad-complex tachycardia cannot be determined, regard it as ventricular tachycardia.

5 Attention to hypoxia, heart failure, acid–base and electrolyte balance, continuing ischaemia, pre-existing bradycardia, and endocrine disorders should not be forgotten in the rush to use anti-arrhythmic drugs.

6 All anti-arrhythmic drugs have disadvantages. Atrial or ventricular pacing, or other electrical techniques should always be considered and will sometimes be preferable.

7 Even in skilled hands in a high-dependency unit, the speed of delivery of a DC shock for ventricular fibrillation can be improved by the use of automated defibrillators.

Introduction

This chapter will encompass the recognition and treatment of arrhythmias that cause either circulatory arrest or a profound fall in cardiac output.

Diagnosis

The correct interpretation of an arrhythmia requires a 'noise-free' ECG, a lead configuration that gives a clear P wave as well as a distinct QRS (leads II and V_1 are best), and a familiarity with the patterns and mechanisms of common rhythm disorders. These ideals may be difficult to achieve during cardiopulmonary arrest.

The diagnosis of tachycardias (rates >100/min) is often more difficult than the diagnosis of bradycardias (rates <60/min). Fast rhythms have a wider range of possible causes, and crowding of the ECG deflections obscures atrial activity. The practical points listed in Box 7.1 are helpful, particularly where the diagnosis is challenging. A more detailed discussion of the recognition of ventricular tachycardia (VT) is presented later in the chapter.

Ventricular fibrillation

Ventricular fibrillation is recognizable as a virtually chaotic record. It may vary from coarse, with large discrete deflections (Fig. 7.1a), to fine (Fig. 7.1b), where it may be difficult to distinguish from asystole. The amplitude setting of a monitor can easily alter the eye's impression of how coarse the rhythm appears.

The treatment is immediate external defibrillation as described in Chapter 2. To recap, the sequence is: 3-shocks-in-a-row (200, 200, and 360 J); then adrenaline; 10 CPR sequences; and then 3 further shocks at 360 J. The loop of adrenaline—CPR—3 shocks is repeated as long as defibrillation is indicated (p. 20).

With a growing recognition that the time to defibrillation is

Box 7.1 ● Practical points that may be helpful in the diagnosis of tachycardias

- A full 12-lead recording is essential for the correct diagnosis of tachycardia, and should be obtained wherever possible.
- Access to previous ECG records can be helpful to define the usual QRS pattern of the patient or to compare earlier episodes of tachycardia.
- Look for atrial activity (distinct P waves, or the rapid deflections of atrial flutter or fibrillation) and its relationship to the QRS complex. Remember that P waves and T waves can overlap; finding P waves needs careful scrutiny.
- Look for any regularity of pattern, even when the trace initially looks chaotic.
- Try to understand the most normal-looking part of the ECG before tackling the more challenging sequences.
- *Sinus tachycardias* of more than 130/minute at rest are uncommon.
- Regular rates of 145–155 per minute with narrow QRS complexes are often due to atrial flutter with 2:1 block.
- Narrow QRS complexes indicate that the arrhythmia is supraventricular (that is, the abnormality is mostly dependent on a mechanism above the division of the bundle of His).
- Broad QRS complexes mean either a ventricular origin or a supraventricular origin with abnormal conduction. The less the pattern is like right-bundle branch-block, the more likely the rhythm is to be of ventricular origin. In ischaemic heart disease regard all broad QRS beats as ventricular in origin until proved otherwise.

critical to the survival from VF, emergency devices have been developed that diagnose and treat this arrhythmia automatically. Two versions exist: (1) the fully automated defibrillator, which on sensing the arrhythmia charges and delivers a shock without operator intervention; and (2) the semi-automatic, or 'advisory' defibrillator (Fig. 7.2), which after rhythm analysis

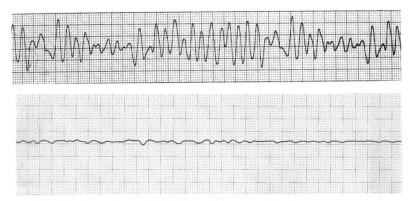

Fig. 7.1 ● Ventricular fibrillation: (a) coarse; (b) fine.

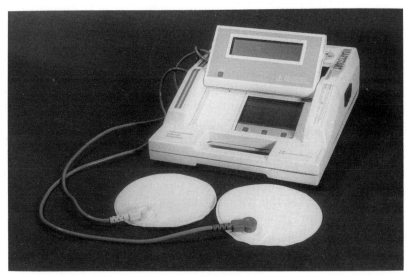

Fig. 7.2 ● An automatic 'advisory' defibrillator.

indicates to the operator that a shock is (or is not) recommended, while leaving her or him to trigger its delivery. The latter version has become the more widely accepted by those most closely involved with resuscitation procedures in practice and by several national advisory authorities. All defibrillators with a diagnostic capability are now known as 'automated defibrillators'.

The diagnostic algorithms used in these devices are remarkably effective, having both a sensitivity and a specificity for ventricular fibrillation of over 95 per cent. In comparison with paramedic crews they perform with equal accuracy, and give a similar rate of successful defibrillation—and they work faster! The availability of these devices in ambulances and in selected areas of a hospital should be considered part of a district resuscitation strategy, and is now a Department of Health recommendation.

Internal defibrillation, using small paddles applied directly to the heart and shocks of up to 20 J, may be indicated when the chest has been opened for internal cardiac massage (p. 27) and ventricular fibrillation proves refractory. The treatment of recurrent ventricular fibrillation or tachycardia by a permanently implanted automatic defibrillator is discussed on p. 136.

In life-threatening emergencies there is no contraindication to the use of external defibrillation in patients with implanted pacemakers or internal automatic defibrillators (AICDs). But if at all possible, defibrillating paddles should be placed as well away from the implanted device; and it should always be assumed that the permanent system is likely to have been damaged by the several thousand volts of the external shock. Even if the capacity of the pacemaker or AICD to deliver an impulse is unaffected, the functions of internal signal detection or programming may well have been destroyed.

Therapy of the patient after successful defibrillation from VF requires prophylaxis against recurrence, using lignocaine as the initial treatment (p. 161), as well as attention to hypoxia, hypokalaemia, magnesium status, ongoing myocardial ischaemia, and heart failure.

Ventricular tachycardia

Ventricular tachycardia (VT) usually originates in a small group of abnormal myocardial cells. It may be associated with an area of infarction or with limited ischaemia due to microemboli in small coronary vessels; it may arise in ventricular muscle that is hypertrophied or myopathic. Cardiac failure, continuing ischaemia, hypokalaemia, reduced tissue magnesium, raised catecholamine levels, and (paradoxically) a slow sinus rate all predispose to the development of VT.

Ventricular tachycardia may be preceded by a number of 'warning' ventricular arrhythmias (Fig. 7.3), although faith in their predictive power has waned since they were first described by Lown in 1968. But the 'higher grade' warning arrhythmias, R-on-T or multiform ectopics and brief runs of VT, are still regarded as sinister, especially if they occur in combination.

Ventricular tachycardia may occur at a wide variety of rates. (If 'VT' occurs at rates of less than 100 per minute the disorder is described as 'idioventricular rhythm'.) In general, the higher the rate the more profound the haemodynamic disturbance. Higher rates are also associated with greater resistance to therapy, easier degeneration to ventricular fibrillation, and poorer long-term outcome. But with good underlying left ventricular function, rates of up to 150 per minute may be surprisingly well tolerated; VT in this setting may be present for hours or even days before medical advice is sought. The patient's clinical state alone may not suffice to differentiate between ventricular tachycardia and supraventricular tachycardia with aberration.

Recognition and differential diagnosis

Ventricular tachycardia—a sequence of repetitive ventricular premature beats—presents as a broad-complex tachycardia arising independently of any underlying atrial activity. The chief differential diagnosis is a supraventricular rhythm, originating above the division of the His bundle but associated with abnormal or 'aberrant' conduction. Such aberration may be part of the patient's usual ECG pattern (seen, for example, in a patient with established left-bundle branch-block who develops rapid atrial fibrillation), or may occur because the conducting system fails at the higher rate demanded of it by the supraventricular tachycardia (SVT). The right-bundle branch is particularly vulnerable in this regard.

Occasionally, a tachycardia arising in the bundle branches themselves rather than in the ventricular myocardium (a 'fas-

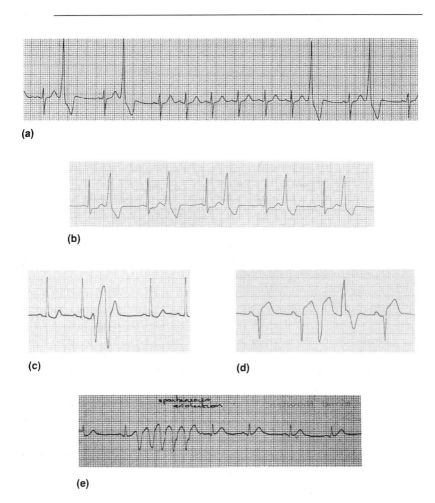

Fig. 7.3 • 'Warning' ventricular arrhythmias of increasing severity:
(a) Frequent single uniform ventricular premature beats.
(b) Coupled ventricular extrasystoles. (c) The R-on-T phenomenon,
in which the R wave of two ventricular premature beats fall on the
T wave of the preceding beat. (See also Fig. 7.3e) (d) Multiform
ventricular premature beats. These may or may not represent a
number of separate foci for the abnormal beats; but they do
indicate markedly increased ventricular excitability. (See also Fig.
5.8) (e) Brief run of ventricular tachycardia beginning with R-on-T
ectopic.

cicular' tachycardia) will mimic true VT; but this differential is less common and less important.

Although the advice may sound repetitive, the value of a 12-lead electrocardiogram in a broad-complex tachycardia cannot be over-emphasized. It allows a full range of leads to capture diagnostic features; it will be useful for comparison with previous or subsequent tracings; and it may be vital for the later management of the patient who requires long-term antitachy-cardia pacing or surgery.

Boxes 7.2 and 7.3 give useful diagnostic clues in the differential diagnosis of a broad-complex tachycardia.

Understanding the activity of the atria is the first step; if the identification of P waves on the ECG is difficult, additional recording techniques may be considered. An oesophageal lead (using a bipolar pacing wire position to lie behind the heart) will clarify the timing of the left atrial deflection, but requires a special pre-amplifier, and may not be well tolerated by the patient.

An intra-atrial electrogram is achieved by positioning a transvenous pacing wire to lie in the high right atrium. By attaching the arm leads of an electrocardiograph to the bipolar wire connections and the leg leads as usual a recording of the standard leads I, II, and III will identify P wave activity as a sharp high-amplitude deflection (Fig. 7.4).

The detailed morphology of the QRS complex, particularly its initial deflection, is also a key feature in the differential

---

Box 7.2 ● Features usually associated with supraventricular tachycardia and aberration

- P waves occur in a one-to-one relation with QRS complexes.
- The pattern recorded will be identical or very similar to that of any pre-existing bundle branch-block.
- An rSR[1] pattern in lead V_1 (typical of right-bundle branch-block) is likely to be present, and a qRS will be recorded in V_6.
- The second beat of the run is usually the most abnormal.

Box 7.3 ● Features pointing to a ventricular tachycardia

- Known ischaemic heart-disease present
- P waves that are independent (an atrial electrogram may be required for confirmation)
- A QRS duration of more than 140 msec if the QRS is normal during sinus rhythm
- The presence of fusion beats. Fusion beats occur as a result of the collision between a normally conducted beat and a beat of ventricular origin. The pattern obtained is usually a clear mixture of the two morphologies (Fig. 7.5)
- The presence of capture beats (occasional beats where a sinus impulse is conducted normally to the ventricle)
- A qR in V_1 (but take care if an anterior infarct is present)
- An Rsr[1] in lead V_1, i.e. a tall initial R wave and a pattern that otherwise resembles right-bundle branch-block (Fig. 7.6)
- A bizarre frontal plane axis, particularly one that gives rise to a strongly positive deflection in aVR (Fig. 7.7); this is a sensitive diagnostic feature
- A QS, rS, or S wave in V_6 (that is, V_6 has little or no R wave)—but beware the mimic of lateral infarction
- Concordant V leads—that is, the QRS deflection is either positive or negative in every lead from V_1 to V_6 (Fig. 7.8).
- Changing wave fronts, as in Torsade de pointes (Fig. 7.9)
- The presence of a QRS wave that is deepest in leads V_4 and V_5 (distinguishable from left-bundle branch-block, in which the deepest QS is in V_1 and V_3)
- An initial deflection that is different from that of conducted beats
- The presence of more than one broad complex morphology on the same recording
- A pattern resembling previously diagnosed VT

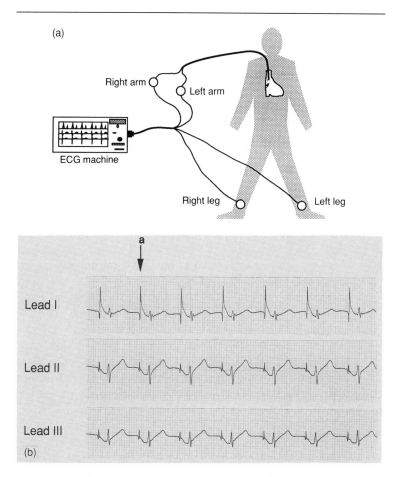

Fig. 7.4 ● Recording an atrial electrogram: (a) The lead connections using a standard electrocardiograph and a bipolar pacing wire in the high right atrium. (b) Leads I, II, and III as recorded by this technique. Atrial activity **a** is shown by a sharp deflection. The QRS activity in 'lead I' is virtually eliminated.

diagnosis of a possible ventricular tachycardia. In VT, a tall initial R wave in aVR and V_1 is a common and helpful finding, and the QRS axis in the limb leads is frequently bizarre. Even with careful ECG evaluation it may prove impossible to understand the mechanism of a broad-complex tachycardia. The golden rule remains—if in doubt, the diagnosis is ventricular.

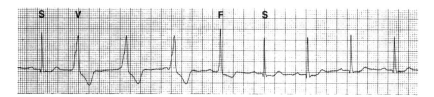

Fig. 7.5 ● Fusion beat. The beat marked F is the result of collision between a ventricular ectopic beat (V) and normal sinus beat (S), giving a mixed pattern. This finding confirms the origin of the broad complex beats as ventricular.

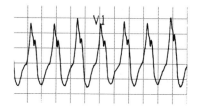

Fig. 7.6 ● The appearance in V_1 of the QRS complex in ventricular tachycardia. The initial R wave is the tallest positive deflection, Rrs[1].

Urgent treatment

Therapy for ventricular tachycardia is directed at conversion to sinus rhythm and the prevention of recurrent attacks (or subsequent ventricular fibrillation). The priorities for treatment will depend on the rate and on the haemodynamic effect of the arrhythmia:

● Pulseless VT (usually with rate greater than 180 per minute or with poor myocardial function) requires immediate treatment as for ventricular fibrillation.
● Ventricular tachycardia with a poor haemodynamic state (usually rapid) is also an indication for urgent DC cardioversion. Unless the haemodynamic state is very poor or is deteriorating rapidly obtain good intravenous access and give shocks synchronized to the R wave as necessary under light

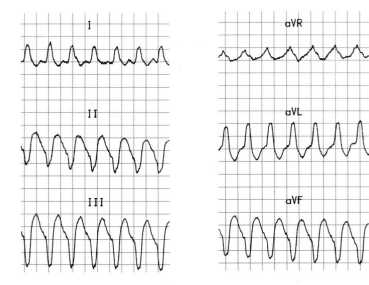

Fig. 7.7 • Ventricular tachycardia reflected in the limb leads. Note the unusual frontal plane axis, with a positive deflection in aVR.

(intravenous) anaesthetic. Begin with 100 J. Energies lower than this may induce ventricular fibrillation.

- Less rapid but sustained VT (rates under 150/min or below) in patients with adverse signs will also require synchronized cardioversion.
- For slower rates, with a good haemodynamic status, or where VT is paroxysmal and recurrent rather than sustained, pharmacological treatment is indicated as the first measure.

Pharmacological therapy

Before using specific suppressant drugs consider the following:

- Is the underlying atrial rate too slow? If so, atropine—or atrial pacing—may increase basic heart rate sufficiently to suppress ectopic ventricular pacemaker activity.
- Is hypokalaemia present? Aim to achieve a potassium level of at least 4 mmol per litre by intravenous infusion.

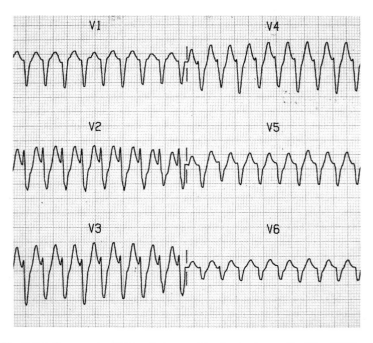

Fig. 7.8 ● Concordant V leads in ventricular tachycardia. The QRS complexes are uniformly negative.

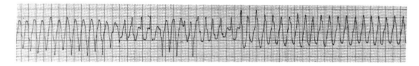

Fig. 7.9 ● Torsade de pointes. A rapid ventricular rhythm with a changing direction of QRS 'points'.

● Is magnesium indicated? Intravenous magnesium sulphate is helpful:
  – for patients with hypokalaemia;
  – for those who have received diuretic treatment before admission;
  – where left ventricular function is impaired; and
  – where underlying conduction defects are present.

- Is treatment required at all? Short runs of asymptomatic VT without haemodynamic disturbance may not require suppressant therapy. Correcting basic heart rate, electrolyte disturbances, heart failure, arterial Po_2 or ischaemia is likely to prove more beneficial than cardio-depressant drugs.
- Is the rhythm Torsade de pointes? The rhythm is characterized by changing wave fronts of ventricular activation (Fig. 7.9). It should be treated by correcting electrolyte disorders (including magnesium) and by increasing the basic heart rate if possible, but *not* by anti-tachycardia drugs. These may make the problem worse.

Anti-arrhythmic drug therapy should start with lignocaine, the agent of first choice for the conversion of ventricular tachycardia and for prophylaxis against recurrent attacks. An initial loading dose of 50 mg is given intravenously over 2 minutes, repeated at 5-minute intervals to a total of 4 doses— provided no serious adverse response occurs. An infusion is started at a rate of 2 mg per minute at a time the first bolus is injected. After 3 hours the infusion rate is reduced to 1.5 mg per minute, and this is continued for the next 24 hours. Doses are reduced in the elderly, in those with hepatic impairment, and where a bradycardia or hypotension are evident.

Further DC shocks may be administered, if required, for sustained VT after lignocaine (and potassium/magnesium, if necessary) has been started. Energies of 100, 200, and then 300 J are recommended.

Subsequent agents used where lignocaine fails will usually be drawn from the following, bearing in mind that drugs have substantial disadvantages as well as benefits in the management of ventricular arrhythmias.

- *Amiodarone*: 300 mg intravenously given over 5–15 minutes, then 600 mg over 1 hour in urgent cases. (Give over a longer period if less urgent.)
- *Procainamide*: 100 mg intravenously given over 5 minutes, with one or two further boluses before the use of an infusion at 3 mg per minute
- *Disopyramide*: 2 mg/kg intravenously given over 20 minutes and repeated over 1 hour.
- *Bretylium tosylate*: 400–500 mg diluted in 5 per cent dextrose infused over 10 minutes.

- *Flecainide*: 2 mg/kg intravenously to a maximum of 150 mg given over 30 minutes.

A suggested algorithm for the treatment of broad-complex tachcardias (Fig. 7.10) has recently been published by the European Resuscitation Council as part of its recommendations on the management of 'peri-arrest arrhythmias' (arrhythmias likely to be encountered before or after a cardiac arrest). An important component of this and the Council's similar algorithms for narrow-complex tachycardias and bradycardias, is advice on when expert help should be sought; but as expert help may not always be available immediately, the most likely pattern for continued management is also shown.

Non-pharmacological treatment

The disadvantages of drug therapy (particularly speed of action, myocardial suppression, and pro-arrhythmic effects) lie behind the increasing tendency for electrical modalities to be used in the management of ventricular tachycardia.

DC shock Rapid ventricular rates with serious haemodynamic disturbance require DC cardioversion. Paddle position is the same as the treatment for ventricular fibrillation, and a shock sequence of 100, 200 and 360 J is recommended. (Ventricular tachycardia will often revert at relatively low energies.) Synchronization of the shock to the R wave is preferable to avoid the shock-on-T phenomenon leading to more rapid ventricular tachycardia or fibrillation. Failure to convert at higher energies indicates the need to repeat the 360 J shock after a bolus of lignocaine.

Pacing techniques Difficulties are encountered when ventricular tachycardia occurs repeatedly in spite of metabolic correction and first-line suppressant therapy. Progression to stronger pharmacological agents may be precluded by myocardial depression—or may also have been found ineffective. Pacing techniques are then a valuable alternative.

Atrial pacing may be a successful prophylactic technique, simply by increasing basic heart rate to suppress the emergence of ectopic rhythms. For this technique to work, AV nodal conduction must be intact; and unless specially shaped wires are used, it may be difficult to achieve atrial pacing that is stable for several hours.

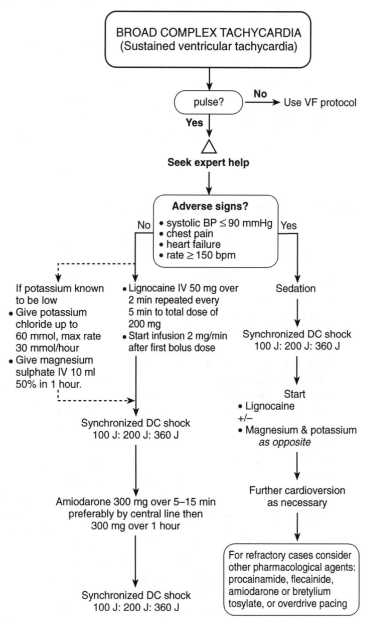

Fig. 7.10 • Flowchart for the treatment of broad-complex tachycardia.

Ventricular pacing has an added advantage in causing myocardial depolarization in a pattern that differs from normal. By this means, overdrive ventricular pacing at a rate only a little above sinus rate may successfully suppress a ventricular tachycardia for several days while other measures are adopted to correct the underlying pathology. Disadvantages include loss of atrial synchronization (with possible adverse haemodynamic effect) and irritation by the pacing wire of the ectopic-producing area near the tricuspid valve.

Ventricular pacing *during* ventricular tachycardia may also be successful in terminating the arrhythmia. Pacing is initiated at a rate above that of the tachycardia, and conversion to sinus rhythm is achieved either by gradually reducing the rate or by suddenly switching off the pacing impulses.

Endocavity cardioversion/defibrillation Internal DC shocks of 1–2 J delivered to the endocardium through temporary transvenous electrodes have occasionally proved of help in the management of recurrent VT. But insertion of the necessarily large (12F) electrodes is difficult, and passage of the wire over the tricuspid valve may itself be arrhythmogenic. Internally delivered shocks are also uncomfortable for the patient.

The implantable defibrillator/cardioverter, introduced clinically in 1980 by Mirowski, now has an established role in the chronic treatment of recurrent life-threatening ventricular tachycardia and fibrillation. It is estimated that well over 10 000 units have been implanted world-wide. The units are inserted into a subcutaneous abdominal pocket, and deliver shocks of 23–37 J to the myocardium through endocavity and/or patch electrodes sewn on to the heart during a limited thoracotomy. Separate sensing electrodes are also required for the automatic diagnosis of the malignant rhythm. Simpler, entirely percutaneous electrode systems are being used increasingly.

These units can dramatically improve the quality and length of life in selected patients: in one series, a 95 per cent survival at three years after implantation was reported, compared with less than 50 per cent for controls. The use of anti-arrhythmic drugs, with their attendant side-effects, can be minimized, or perhaps avoided completely, further improving the enjoyment of life. But the units are expensive (£9000–£13 000); their insertion and testing is demanding (though with very low operative mortality); and they unavoidably call for associated electrophysiological expertise. New devices often include a facility for pacing as well as cardioversion, since deaths in a number of patients in whom they have been implanted are now known to be due to asystole rather than refractory ventricular arrhythmias.

The presence of an implanted automatic defibrillator should not influence the conduct of the recommended emergency measures for treating ventricular fibrillation and tachycardia.

Supraventricular tachycardia

'Supraventricular tachycardia' (SVT) encompasses any tachycardia caused by an abnormal mechanism above the division of the His bundle. The commonest form of SVT (Fig. 7.11) depends on a re-entry circuit where impulses pass back from the ventricle to the atrium through an abnormal pathway, and then forward again into the ventricle via the AV node and conducting system (Fig. 7.12). But its definition also strictly includes atrial flutter and fibrillation, atrial ectopic tachycardia, multifocal atrial tachycardia, and ectopic junctional rhythms. The QRS complexes in all forms of supraventricular tachycardia are narrow—unless pre-existing bundle branch-block is present or aberration occurs because of an increased heart rate, giving rise to the alternative term for these arrhythmias: 'narrow-complex tachycardias'.

It is uncommon for SVT to cause profound circulatory collapse. Rates are usually under 200 per minute, and many

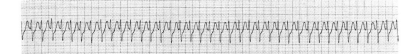

Fig. 7.11 ● A typical supraventricular tachycardia with narrow QRS complexes.

patients are young or middle aged, with no other cardiac disease. But attacks may compromise the circulation if they are prolonged and either ventricular rates are unusually high (>250/min), or the arrhythmia is superimposed on underlying coronary, valvular, or myocardial disease. The former occurs where AV conduction is enhanced—usually by an abnormal pathway bypassing the delay circuits of the AV node. Rates in these conditions may exceed 300 per minute. In a few cases of Wolff–Parkinson–White (WPW) syndrome, atrial fibrillation may result in dangerously rapid ventricular rates (Fig. 7.13).

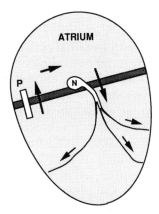

Fig. 7.12 • The re-entry mechanism for common forms of supraventricular tachycardia. Conduction passes down the AV node (N), and then retrogradely through a bypass pathway (P) to reactivate the atrium and the AV node.

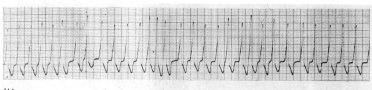

V4 —→

Fig. 7.13 • Rapid atrial fibrillation in the Wolff–Parkinson–White syndrome, giving an alarmingly high ventricular rate.

In the treatment of narrow-complex tachycardias, vagal manoeuvres (in particular a Valsalva manoeuvre or carotid sinus massage) may be effective; but in the context of resuscitation the hazards must be emphasized. In particular, intense vagal stimulation that causes a sudden bradycardia may trigger ventricular fibrillation in the presence of acute myocardial ischaemia. Elderly patients are also vulnerable to carotid plaque rupture with cerebrovascular complications.

The pharmacological treatment of choice for regular supraventricular tachycardias is adenosine (p. 174). Although this causes unpleasant side-effects (nausea, flushing, and chest discomfort), these are brief and well tolerated, particularly if the patient is informed of their nature and duration before the injection is given. Use a small initial dose of 3 mg. This will be effective in only a minority of cases, but increments can be given every one to two minutes, with at least two injections of 12 mg if necessary. If adenosine is not successful in establishing a satisfactory rhythm, or if atrial fibrillation is present at a rate greater than 130 beats per minute, expert help should be sought. At this point, management will depend on whether or not adverse clinical signs are present, the determinants being similar to those for broad-complex tachycardia.

If adverse signs *are* present, the patient should be sedated and treated by synchronized DC shock. If this is unsuccessful, it should be repeated after the adminstration of intravenous amiodarone as an initial slow injection followed by an infusion; depending upon the need for urgency, up to an hour may elapse before further shocks are attempted.

In the absence of adverse signs, no single recommendation for drug therapy can be made because of different traditions of treatment between and within the European countries. The suggestions encompassed by the ERC's algorithm include a short-acting beta blocker such as esmolol, digoxin, verapamil, and amiodarone. Overdrive pacing may also be successful.

A 50 J shock may be sufficient to convert atrial flutter to sinus rhythm. (Atrial flutter commonly presents with 2:1 block, giving a regular pathological tachycardia at 150 per minute.) But most SVT's will require 100 J or more.

Because of its common presentation, special mention will be made of atrial fibrillation. Like ventricular tachycardia, atrial fibrillation may present with a wide variety of ventricular rates. Aberrant conduction may occur, and the baseline may reveal 'fine' or 'coarse' deflections (Fig. 7.14). Treatment depends on the haemodynamic disturbance caused. Rates under 100 per minute usually require no treatment. Higher rates with no haemodynamic impairment respond to intravenous digoxin. The regimen can be digoxin 500 μg in 100 ml 5 per cent dextrose given over 30 minutes repeated over 1 hour, or ouabain 1 mg in 100–200 ml 5 per cent dextrose given over 1 hour. With haemodynamic compromise, recent unstable myocardial ischaemia, or infarction, a synchronized DC shock is appropriate, beginning at 100 J. But take care if AF has been present for longer than about 6 hours: restoration of sinus rhythm occasionally results in arterial embolization, and the prudent use of digoxin and anticoagulants may be preferable.

Paroxysmal atrial fibrillation is usually well controlled by amiodarone (given intravenously in stubborn cases); but this drug is not without its drawbacks. Its use is recommended where digoxin and/or beta blockers fail or cannot be used, or

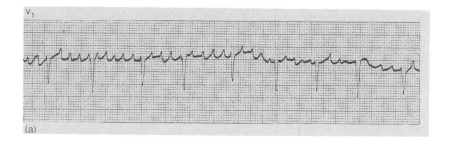

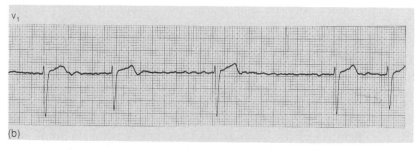

Fig. 7.14 ● Atrial fibrillation: (a) coarse; (b) fine.

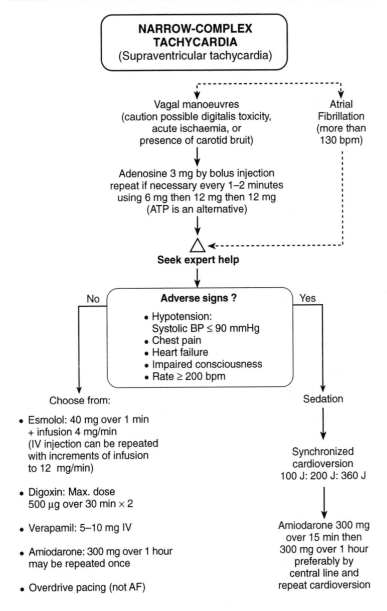

Fig. 7.15 ● Flowchart for the management of narrow-complex tachycardia.

where the underlying condition is self-limiting (e.g. pericarditis after cardiac surgery or myocardial infarction).

Finally, remember to check the thyroid-function tests in 'unexplained' atrial fibrillation, especially in the elderly. The arrhythmia may be their only symptom of thyrotoxicosis. The flowchart for the treatment of narrow-complex tachycardias, including atrial fibrillation is shown in Fig. 7.15.

Bradycardia and asystole

Clinical setting

A pathological bradycardia may be the result of conducting system disease, inferior myocardial infarction, or both, and may be worsened by the presence of beta blocking or other depressant drugs. In acute ischaemic syndromes a modest bradycardia is advantageous in reducing oxygen consumption; but more serious slowing predisposes to ventricular arrhythmias and reduced cardiac output.

In inferior infarction, first-degree AV block and second-degree Wencheback AV block (Fig. 7.16) are common, and usually need no treatment. But if in anterior myocardial infarction there is evidence of a progressive conduction disorder below the AV node the risk of asystole is high. Such evidence would include RBBB with LAD and a lengthening PR interval or a dropped P wave—'Mobitz II block' (Fig. 7.17). The insertion of a prophylactic pacing wire is recommended if these signs are observed.

Established asystole from cardiac causes (especially when P waves are absent) usually indicates extensive muscle damage—although it can follow repeated DC shocks and intense anti-arrhythmic therapy. Profound bradycardia and asystole may also follow severe hypoxia or hypothermia (see p. 41) or the massive parasympathetic outflow of facial injury or near-drowning. Treatment here should be directed initially to the underlying pathology.

Asystole may be difficult to differentiate from fine ventricular fibrillation (see p. 123); in which case it should be treated as VF. Asystole with P waves has a better chance for recovery than 'straight-line' asystole, which, if persistent for more than a minute, is almost invariably fatal.

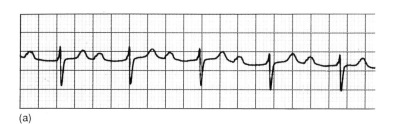

(a)

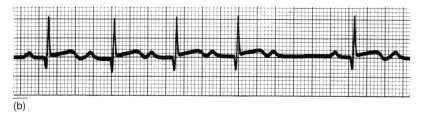

(b)

Fig. 7.16 ● AV block. (a) first-degree—prolonged PR interval. (b) second-degree Wenckeback block. The PR interval gradually lengthens until, for one beat, complete failure of AV conduction occurs.

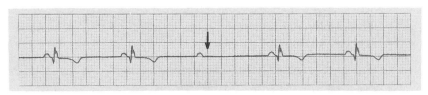

Fig. 7.17 ● Mobitz II AV block. Conduction below the AV node fails abruptly (arrow) without gradual lengthening of the PR interval. There may be evidence of conduction system impairment in the remainder of the record (e.g. left-axis deviation and right-bundle branch-block).

Pharmacological therapy

The treatment of a bradycardia depends first on whether it is likely to be associated with a risk of asystole and secondly—if not—whether any adverse signs are present (Fig. 7.18).

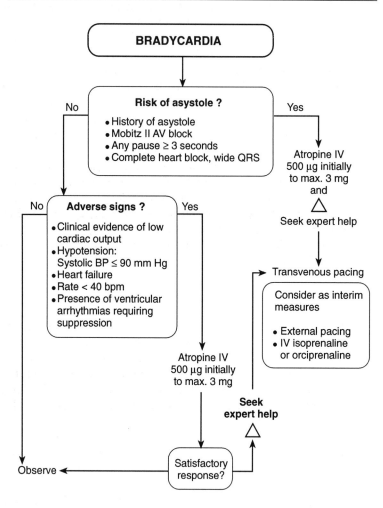

Fig. 7.18 • Flowchart for the management of bradycardia.

Treatment with atropine in doses up to 3 mg intravenously is indicated as initial therapy for a high-risk haemodynamically significant bradycardia with narrow QRS complexes, especially where the underlying mechanism is thought to be high parasympathetic tone or acute inferior myocardial infarction.

In asystole, adrenaline is the first drug of choice, at a dose of 1 mg delivered as centrally as possible. Chest compression should be given for one minute to allow a full drug effect. In a patient in profound bradycardia or asystole with P waves an isoprenaline infusion of 1–4 µg per minute may also sustain a spontaneous cardiac rhythm until more definitive procedures can be implemented. Dilute 2 mg of isoprenaline in 500 ml 5 per cent dextrose; this gives a concentration of 4 µg/ml.

The contribution of calcium chloride to recovery from asystole or electromechanical dissociation is now questioned. Though electromechanical coupling requires calcium ions, profound myocardial ischaemia causes a catastrophic increase in intracellular calcium. Calcium chloride should be considered only for patients with asystole or electromechanical dissociation associated with hypocalaemia, or where calcium-channel blocking drugs may have contributed to cardiac depression.

Non-pharmacological treatment

Temporary transvenous ventricular pacing is indicated in any patient with transient or threatened asystole or a haemodynamically significant bradycardia unresponsive to drugs. Other definite indications include complete heart-block associated with anterior infarction; a slow escape rhythm (less than 40 per minute); wide QRS complexes; a low blood pressure; or syncope.

The patient may need support until preparation of the appropriate equipment with atropine, isoprenaline, or adrenaline, supplemented, if necessary, by cardiopulmonary resuscitation.

Unipolar ventricular stimulation is advisable for patients after acute myocardial infarction; and antibiotics should be used to cover any rapid procedure where aseptic precautions have been breached.

Inserting a transvenous wire during cardiopulmonary resuscitation is difficult. It also requires a skilled operator and X-ray screening facilities. For this reason external 'transcutaneous' pacing devices have again become fashionable (Fig. 7.19). These deliver a 20–200-milliamp transcutaneous pulse several milliseconds long through large-diameter adhesive

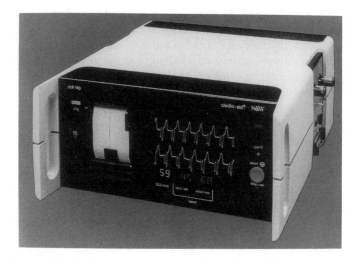

Fig. 7.19 • A device to deliver transcutaneous pacing stimuli for emergency cardiac support.

electrodes; and they can achieve cardiac capture if the heart has not lost all evidence of spontaneous electrical activity. Unfortunately, they can cause discomfort to the patient because of the stimulation of nerve endings and skeletal muscle in the chest wall. Their use is primarily to gain time in a critical phase of collapse, before more definitive treatment can be applied.

Other devices have been designed for temporary pacing in the emergency situation. Transoesophageal pacing will readily stimulate the left atrium through the oesophageal wall; but it cannot overcome atrio-ventricular block, and is remote from the ventricle. Ventricular stimulation via an electrode inserted through the chest wall ('transthoracic pacing') suffers the disadvantage of seriously interfering with chest compression. This is especially true of an approach to the heart through a left parasternal intercostal space—a position that also threatens transection of the left anterior descending coronary artery. The rule appears to be that if pacing is going to be effective then there is time to insert a conventional transvenous system.

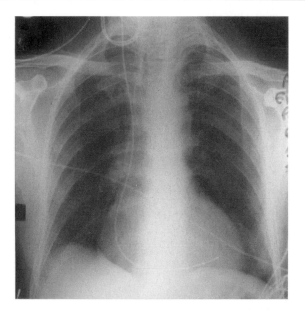

Fig. 7.20 ● X-ray of a pacing wire.

'Last-ditch' rescue by more heroic approaches is usually doomed by the underlying pathology.

Further reading

1. Advanced Cardiac Life Support Committee of the European Resuscitation Council (1994). Management of peri-arrest arrhythmias. *Resuscitation*, **28**, 151–9.

2. Aronson, J. K. (1985). Cardiac arrhythmias: theory and practice. *British Medical Journal*, **290**, 487–8.

3. Bennett, D. H. (1985). *Cardiac arrhythmias, Practical notes on interpretation and treatment*, (2nd edn). John Wright, Bristol.

4. Dancy, M., Camm, A. J., and Ward, D. (1985). Misdiagnosis of chronic recurrent ventricular tachycardia. *Lancet*, **ii**, 320–3.

5. Julian, D. G. (1983). Disorders of rate, rhythm and condition. Chapter 4 in *Concise medical text books: cardiology*, pp. 49–78. Baillière Tindall, London.

6. Schamroth, L. (1980). *The disorders of cardiac rhythm.* Blackwell, Oxford.
7. Ward, D. E. and Camm, A. J. (1987). *Clinical electrophysiology of the heart.* Edward Arnold, London.

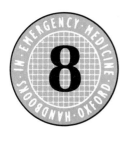

CHAPTER 8

Biochemistry and pharmacology of cardiac arrest

149

Key points in the biochemistry and pharmacology of cardiac arrest

1 The primary metabolic derangements following cardiac arrest are a profound hypoxia and an acidosis derived from both carbon dioxide retention and an increased production of lactic acid.

2 Effective cardiopulmonary resuscitation improves the biochemical profile of arterial blood but venous blood, which may better represent tissue status, remains profoundly desaturated, with a progressive hypercarbic acidosis.

3 Intravenous sodium bicarbonate may worsen the acid–base disturbance of a cardiac arrest. It should be given either late in a resuscitation attempt (>10 minutes) after effective ventilation is well established, or when a severe pre-existing acidosis exists.

4 Cardiac arrest is also attended by a marked rise in catecholamines, adrenal steroids, blood sugar, and antidiuretic hormone (ADH), as well as a fall in plasma potassium.

5 Adrenaline given during cardiac arrest improves cerebral and myocardial blood flow, chiefly through receptor-mediated peripheral vasoconstriction. Other catecholamines show no consistent advantage, and isolated β stimulants are detrimental.

6 The routine use of lignocaine after myocardial infarction is not recommended. It remains the second-line drug for treating ventricular fibrillation and for recurrent ventricular tachycardia.

7 Atropine is best used where excessive vagal tone may be contributing to the patient's collapse.

8 Most drugs used to treat or suppress tachy-arrhythmias also depress myocardial function. They often have other unwanted actions, and may occasionally trigger a worsened arrhythmia ('pro-arrhythmic effect').

9 Magnesium therapy should be considered for all ventricular arrhythmias requiring urgent treatment, particularly if the plasma potassium is low.

Biochemical derangements in circulatory arrest

Introduction

The biochemical derangements associated with cardiac arrest are determined partly by the clinical setting in which the arrest occurred, and partly by the effects of circulatory stand-still whatever the cause. For example, cardiac arrest following a period of profound hypoxia may be accompanied by a metabolic acidosis, whereas when ventilation has been sup-pressed (stroke, drugs) or obstructed (choking, trauma, drown-ing), the picture will be complicated by a prior respiratory acidosis with a raised P_{CO_2}.

Pain or fear in the pre-arrest period will trigger a surge in autonomic activity, with both cholinergic and adrenergic effects; potassium and magnesium may have been depleted by chronic diuretic therapy, and alcohol, drugs, or carbon monoxide poisoning will bring their own specific changes to the metabolic milieu of a life-threatening collapse.

But many patients, particularly those suffering unheralded cardiac arrest, have a normal acid–base and biochemical pro-file until the effects of circulatory standstill supervene. These effects are summarized in Box 8.1. The principal biochemical abnormalities seen after cardiac arrest result from the reten-tion of carbon dioxide and an accumulation of the acid prod-ucts of anaerobic metabolism following tissue hypoxia.

Box 8.1 ● Main biochemical derangements following cardiac arrest

- Hypoxia
- Carbon dioxide retention
- Increased production of metabolic acid (lactate)
- Marked elevation of catecholamines
- Increase in adrenocortical steroids
- Rise in plasma antidiuretic hormone (ADH)

Hypoxia

After primary cardiac arrest oxygen tension is preserved for a brief period, but failure of normal pulmonary ventilation and perfusion soon results in a fall in arterial Po_2. Moreover, a rapidly developing respiratory acidosis will shift the haemoglobin oxygen-dissociation curve so that saturation is more difficult to achieve than normal. Mixed venous blood, even during satisfactory chest compression, is severely desaturated. Competently applied cardiopulmonary resuscitation (CPR)—with high levels of inspired oxygen—is essential to correct the hypoxic state.

Acid–base balance

Physiological buffer systems exist to maintain the pH of the blood as close to normal as possible (pH 7.4, [H+] = 40 nmol/l). Plasma-based buffer systems are the most rapidly responsive, and include plasma proteins (particularly albumin), haemoglobin, phosphate, ammonium, and—of special importance in cardiac arrest—the bicarbonate–carbonic acid system. The equation for this reaction is:

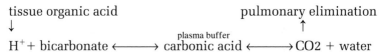

tissue organic acid   pulmonary elimination
↓   ↑
                                    plasma buffer
H^+ + bicarbonate ⟷ carbonic acid ⟷ CO2 + water

For a normal plasma pH, bicarbonate and carbonic acid exist in a 20:1 ratio. This ratio holds the key to pH control.

In cardiopulmonary arrest, extracellular hydrogen ion concentration increases from failure of elimination of CO_2 (through lack of pulmonary perfusion and ventilation), and from the accumulation of organic acid. Since the production of acid (mainly lactate) by anaerobic metabolism is slow,

---

Box 8.2 ● Some important effects of acidosis

- Reduced myocardial contractility
- Reduced automaticity of pacemaker cells
- Decreased threshold for ventricular fibrillation
- Reduced chronotropic and vasopressor action of catecholamines

shifts in CO_2 are considerably more important. Intracellular P_{CO_2} rises more abruptly than carbonic acid levels in the blood. The resulting fall in intracellular pH impedes cellular metabolism, with important consequences (Box 8.2).

Animal and human studies have shown that although arteriovenous differences in pH, P_{CO_2}, and bicarbonate are normally small (Box 8.3), cardiac arrest and subsequent CPR causes a dramatic divergence in acid–base status between the arterial and venous circulations (Fig. 8.1). Mixed venous blood (thought to represent tissue metabolism more accurately than arterial blood) becomes progressively more acidotic, with a rising P_{CO_2}. Studies of regional circulation also suggest that the myocardium and the brain both suffer a more intense acidosis than even a mixed venous sample reflects.

Correction of arterial pH and P_{CO_2} is usually possible with well-performed resuscitation. During CPR, a combination of

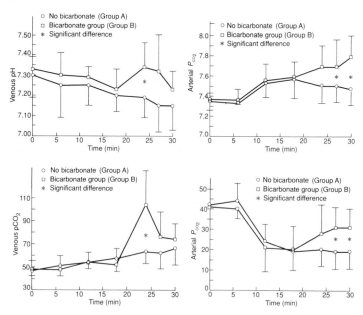

Fig. 8.1 ● Changes in atrial and venous pH and P_{CO_2} following cardiac arrest in experimental dogs.

Box 8.3 ● Normal arterial and venous concentrations of pH, P_{CO_2}, P_{O_2}, and bicarbonate

	Arterial	Venous
pH	7.35–7.45	7.31–7.41
P_{CO_2} (mmHg)	35–45	40–50
P_{CO_2} (mmHg)	90–100	30–40
HCO_3 (mEq/1)	24–28	24–28

---

slow pulmonary flow and assisted hyperventilation allows extensive clearing of the high CO_2 levels presented to the lungs by the venous blood. Indeed the result of CPR is often that arterial P_{CO_2} falls, and its pH rises into an alkalotic range (Fig. 8.1). Venous blood, however, shows an increasing hypercarbic acidosis. Although this is usually termed a 'respiratory acidosis', the rise in venous P_{CO_2} and concomitant fall in pH have a progressively important metabolic drive from the increased production of lactate and CO_2 during anaerobic metabolism.

If arterial gases remain seriously acidotic, inadequate ventilation and then inadequate circulatory support is likely to be the cause. (Figure 8.2 provides a helpful nomogram for the interpretation of acid–base status from arterial blood-gas analysis.) The biochemical profile of arterial blood favouring a successful outcome from CPR is shown in Box 8.4.

Box 8.4 ● Biochemical profile of arterial blood that favours a successful outcome from CPR

pH	7.25–7.55
P_{CO_2}	Value not critical
Bicarbonate	21–35 mEq/l
Lactate	<6.5 mmol/l
Sodium	121–145 mEq/l
Potassium	3.5–5.6 mEq/l
Osmolality	280–350 osmol

Values outside these ranges are associated with a sharp decline in survival.

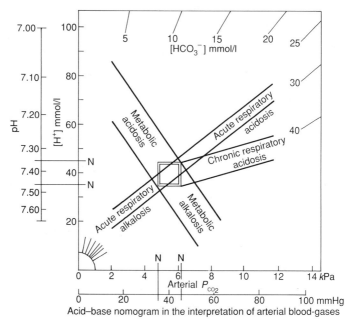

Fig. 8.2 ● A helpful acid–base nomogram for the interpretation of blood gases.

The use of sodium bicarbonate Sodium bicarbonate was once recommended for early use in the correction of acidosis during cardiac arrest. It was assumed that organic acid produced by anaerobic metabolism was chiefly responsible for the change in blood pH, and that this could best be buffered with additional HCO_3^- ions. But *in vivo*, solutions of sodium bicarbonate release large quantities of carbon dioxide into the blood by driving the equation on p. 153 towards the right. Infused intravenously, bicarbonate worsens the existing hypercarbic state (Fig. 8.1). Moreover, released carbon dioxide diffuses more rapidly into cells than the bicarbonate ion, resulting in increasing intracellular acidosis and worsening cellular function. The brain may be especially at risk, since the blood–brain barrier is more readily crossed by carbon dioxide than by bicarbonate ions, resulting in a depression of higher functions that may contribute to post-resuscitation confusion and restlessness. Intracellular acidosis in the heart leads to reduced contractility, and contributes to electrome-chanical dissociation.

Other potentially damaging effects of sodium bicarbonate are hyperosmolality and sodium overload (Box 8.5). For these reasons, bicarbonate administration has been relegated to a stage late in the arrest procedure, after a minimum of 10 minutes of full cardiopulmonary support. Also, before using bicarbonate, effective ventilation via an endotracheal tube should be established to ensure adequate elimination of carbon dioxide. Rarely, however, the use of bicarbonate may be indicated earlier in an arrest, when the patient is known to have a severe pre-existing metabolic acidosis (an adverse feature for prognosis). Other buffering agents, such as carbicarb, seem to offer no practical advantage over sodium bicarbonate and have not gained the popularity of use that might have been predicted from their theoretical benefits.

Box 8.5 • Potential adverse effects of sodium bicarbonate therapy during cardiac arrest

- Arterial metabolic alkalosis
- Hypokalaemia
- Hypocalcaemia
- Reduced efficacy of catecholamines
- Hypernatraemia
- Tighter haemoglobin–oxygen binding
- Hyperosmolality
- Intracellular acidosis
- Venus hypercarbic acidosis

Catecholamines

Acute myocardial infarction and cardiac arrest are attended by a marked outpouring of adrenaline from the adrenal medulla and of noradrenaline from sympathetic nerve terminals. In both asystole and ventricular fibrillation, levels of plasma catecholamine, including dopamine, rise far higher than in any other condition. Moreover, release of catecholamines within the myocardium during infarction or cardiac arrest predisposes both to persistent arrhythmias and to patchy myocardial necrosis.

The effects of adrenergic hormones occur through the stimulation of two general classes of receptor, α and β. Both classes have two subtypes (α_1, α_2, β_1, β_2)—although for this discussion the α receptors need not be differentiated. Table 8.1 shows the physiological effect of activating the different receptor types, and their responsiveness to stimulation by three important catecholamines.

The physiological effects of high catecholamine levels at the onset of a cardiac arrest have not been fully explored. An initial attempt at maintaining peripheral resistance with a redistribution of vessel capacitance seems likely; but this may be short lived. A shift of potassium from plasma to skeletal muscle cells, and an elevation in blood sugar, also seem to follow the catecholamine rise, although these changes may have additional causes. It is evident, however, that in spite of high endogenous levels, administered catecholamines still have a beneficial effect in the management of cardiac arrest (p. 22).

Other metabolic changes

A wide variety of other cellular and extracellular metabolic changes occur after cardiopulmonary arrest. All of the responses of severe shock are seen, including an outpouring of adrenal steroids, an elevation of blood sugar (perhaps adversely affecting cerebral outcome), alterations in haematological variables, and an increase in ADH. These may supplement any underlying pathology, opposing the chances of successful resuscitation.

Table 8.1 • Physiological effects of adrenergic receptor stimulation and the activity of catecholamines on different receptor types

	α receptors Vasoconstriction	β receptors ↑ Heart rate ↑ Contractility ↑ Excitability	$\beta2$ receptors Vasodilation ↓ Bronchial tone Glycogenolysis
Adrenaline	+ +	+ +	+
Noradrenaline	+ + +	±	±
Isoprenaline	±	+ + +	+ + +

First-line drugs in cardiac arrest

Oxygen

Arterial hypoxaemia accompanies circulatory standstill or results from a variety of causes that precede cardiac arrest. Hypoxia compromises contractility and the electrical stability of myocardial cells, ultimately leading to cell death. Hypoxia also causes increased sympathetic and vagal activity. Enhanced vagal tone appears, at least in the short term, to contribute more to electrical instability than the adrenergic response—in spite of the increase in free intramyocardial catecholamines that results from hypoxaemia.

Oxygen therapy is correctly prescribed as routine in any presentation of shock or circulatory arrest. An effective method for delivery should be ensured—by well-fitting mask or by endotracheal tube. No hazard will ensue from delivering as high an oxygen concentration as is possible during circulatory arrest. The challenge is usually to raise the arterial P_{O_2} sufficiently.

Adrenaline

Adrenaline is a powerful catecholamine with both α and β effects (Table 8.1). Its benefit in cardiac arrest has been known since 1906, when Crile and Dolley showed a markedly improved survival in experimental dogs by the addition of an adrenaline infusion to artificial ventilation and cardiac massage.

The mechanism of action of adrenaline in cardiac arrest is only partially understood; conflicting data exist about the pharmacological effects and appropriate dose of adrenaline and other catecholamines in this condition. Adrenaline's prime action as a pressor agent is mediated through its α effects on peripheral arterioles, although a β_2 effect is also considered by some to be important in its role of improving cerebral capillary flow.

Even during successful CPR, cerebral and myocardial perfusion are a fraction of normal (Fig. 8.3). Both depend on the aortic diastolic pressure (ADP) that occurs during the relaxation phase of chest compression. Adrenaline undoubtedly

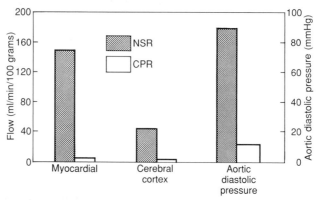

Fig. 8.3 • Myocardial and cerebral blood flow and aortic pressure during cardiopulmonary resuscitation (CPR). Values in normal sinus rhythm (NSR) are shown for comparison.

augments ADP by peripheral vasoconstriction, an effect that gains importance progressively during a resuscitation procedure. Some animal studies suggest that α-mediated effects are also responsible for increasing the chances of successful defibrillation.

In health, β effects cause an increase in sinus rate, the excitability of myocardial cells, conduction velocity, and contractility, and the emergence of subsidiary pacemakers. β_1 stimulation in cardiac arrest has been shown to affect the amplitude and frequency of a ventricular fibrillatory wave form, but probably not to influence the chances of defibrillation or the overall success of a resuscitation attempt.

The dose of adrenaline in cardiac arrest is 1 mg, given as centrally as possible. Absorption via the endotracheal route has been reported to be as little as a tenth as effective as when a central vein is used, even if the dose is doubled. No benefits have been shown from the use of high-dose adrenaline up to 10 mg. Repeated doses are suggested every 2 to 3 minutes during a prolonged arrest to help counteract vascular collapse.

The unwanted effects of adrenaline are an excessive tachycardia, with the metabolic expense of an increased mycardial oxygen requirement. Adrenaline may occasionally be unhelpful in the malignant vicious circle of:

VF–DC shock–asystole–adrenaline–VF–DC
shock–asystole– more adrenaline–VF.

The use of other catecholamines in cardiac arrest has been explored, but none emerge as superior to adrenaline. Agents with a pure β effect (primarily isoprenaline) appear detrimental; and in spite of a theoretical value of pure α stimulation, methoxamine, phenylamine, dopamine, and even noradrenaline fail to show a consistent advantage.

Lignocaine

Lignocaine reduces the excitability of myocardial cells, with a greater effect in ischaemic than in normal tissue. It successfully suppresses ventricular ectopic rhythms, and raises the threshold for ventricular fibrillation (that is, it reduces the readiness with which VF will occur). These properties provide a rationale for its prophylactic use against recurrent malignant ventricular arrhythmias; but give no justification for postulating any beneficial action in established VT or VF.

No convincing evidence exists that lignocaine aids the electrical conversion of VF to sinus rhythm. Indeed, experimentally, lignocaine increases the energy required for defibrillation. The apparent benefit of lignocaine in a VF arrest may be due to the chance success of one further shock irrespective of drug treatment, or to its action in preventing the almost instant recurrence of ventricular fibrillation after a few (perhaps unnoticed) beats of a co-ordinated rhythm that have resulted from a successful shock.

The use of lignocaine routinely after acute myocardial infarction is no longer recommended. Although it successfully reduces both ventricular ectopic activity (a presumed prelude to VF) and the incidence of ventricular fibrillation itself, its beneficial action is counterbalanced by an increased incidence of myocardial depression and asystole. Trials have failed to show any overall reduction in mortality.

Lignocaine remains the first-line drug, however, for:

- suppressing the more aggressive forms of ventricular ectopy during myocardial ischaemia/infarction;
- the conversion or prevention of recurrent ventricular tachycardia;

- the management of refractory VF (p. 00); and
- prophylaxis after successful defibrillation.

For urgent cases the loading dose is 100 mg intravenously (given slowly as two doses of 50 mg), repeated in 15 minutes. For less urgent cases it is preferable to give the total 200 mg as four equal (50 mg) amounts at 5-minute intervals, each injected over about 2 minutes. These schedules reflect the need to avoid an initially high plasma level, with the attendant risk of myocardial suppression.

Following the loading dose, a lignocaine infusion should be started. Use 3 mg/min for 3 hours, then 1.5 mg/min thereafter. If the infusion needs to be continued beyond 24 hours, reduce the rate to 0.75 mg/min. The decreasing dose schedule is recommended because lignocaine gradually depresses its own hepatic metabolism. With a lengthening half-life, progressively less infusate is necessary to maintain an adequate therapeutic effect.

The suggested regimen should readily achieve a steady plasma level in the therapeutic range 1.5–6.0 $\mu g/ml$. Doses should usually be reduced for patients on beta blockers, those in overt heart failure, those with hepatic congestion or disease, those whose sinus rate is already depressed, or those who are unconscious. Lignocaine is less effective by the intramuscular route, and is inactive by mouth. (A drug that mimics the therapeutic profile of lignocaine, but is effective orally, is mexiletine.)

The most important side-effects of lignocaine need re-emphasis. They are listed in Box 8.6. Unfortunately, patients with more serious arrhythmias are the most likely to exhibit these effects though halting the infusion will usually allow a quick, spontaneous recovery.

Box 8.6 • Important adverse cardiovascular effects of lignocaine

- Falling heart rate
- Falling blood pressure
- Myocardial depression
- Greater resistance to defibrillation

Atropine

Atropine opposes the effects of the vagus. It increases sinus rate, and both conduction and automaticity (the rate of spontaneous firing) of the AV node. Vagal depression of atrial and ventricular muscle may also be opposed.

The use of atropine in CPR is limited. For 'true' asystole and electromechanical dissociation, adrenaline takes precedence over atropine because of the advantages of its α effects on vasomotor tone. Occasionally, heightened parasympathetic activity can produce a severe 'braking' effect on the heart. Asystole from intense vagal discharge may occur following facial trauma or from immersion in cold water (the 'diving reflex'). The vagolytic action of atropine is appropriate for these conditions; but the circumstances and time-window for its use are inevitably limited. For other causes of asystole, and when administered with any delay at all, atropine is a very second best to adrenaline.

Atropine is valuable in the face of excessive parasympathetic activity associated with inferior myocardial infarction or reperfusion. Raising the heart rate by enhancing the activity of the SA or AV nodes will reduce the chance of escape ventricular arrhythmias and improve haemodynamic status. An effect on vasomotor tone may also be helpful. The dose is 0.25 mg intravenously followed by further boluses of 0.25–0.5 mg as necessary. Doses of more than 1.5 mg are rarely required.

The unwanted effects of atropine include excessive tachycardia, urinary retention, failure of visual accommodation, and an unwelcome dry mouth. Confusion and restlessness may occur in the elderly, particularly at higher doses.

Bretylium tosylate

Bretylium is a unique drug, with direct and indirect modes of action. Its direct effect on the myocardium—which is poorly understood—raises the threshold to ventricular fibrillation in a similar manner to lignocaine. It prolongs refractory period to a greater degree in normal tissue than in ischaemic or infarcting myocardium, and may therefore prevent micro-re-entry in an ischaemic zone. It appears to have no overall effect on defibrillation threshold (the readiness of a DC shock to restore sinus rhythm).

Bretylium's indirect effect comprises an initial *stimulation* of adrenergic neurones, lasting about 20 minutes, and then an adrenergic *blockade* which peaks some 45–60 minutes later. In addition, bretylium blocks the uptake of noradrenaline into adrenergic nerve terminals. The early adrenergic stimulation may cause transiently improved conduction, and this may contribute to the drug's anti-arrhythmic effect.

The use of bretylium should be considered when electrical countershock plus adrenaline and lignocaine has failed to convert ventricular fibrillation, or where recurrent VF or pulseless ventricular tachycardia occurs in spite of other therapies.

The dose of bretylium is 400 or 500 mg diluted in 5 per cent dextrose given over 10 minutes. Faster use is allowed if necessary—even as a bolus. Bretylium may take 20 minutes to be effective, partly because of its biphasic effect on the adrenergic system. The dose may be repeated after 20 minutes, and again after 1–2 hours if necessary, provided there is no undue cardiac depression, Bretylium can also be used as a maintenance infusion at 1–2 mg/min.

Hypotension may occur as a result of bretylium therapy but is usually transient, and depends partly on peripheral vasodilatation; if it occurs, lay the patient flat, and consider cautious expansion of plasma volume provided there is no significant left ventricular failure.

Anti-tachycardia drugs

Mechanisms of action and classification

Anti-tachycardia drugs, including the already discussed lignocaine and bretylium, suppress the formation of cardiac impulses, or their conduction, or both. In this they mirror the two main mechanisms for a pathological tachycardia:

- increased or triggered automaticity (abnormal impulse formation); and
- re-entry by abnormal conduction through an extra pathway.

The latter may be formed by a myocardial bridge across the AV ring, causing a supraventricular tachycardia (Chapter 7,

p. 138); whereas in ventricular tachycardia the abnormal pathway is often through short intramyocardial circuits involving terminal Purkinje fibres and ischaemic myocardial cells (Fig. 8.4).

The detailed mechanisms by which anti-arrhythmic drugs exert their effect vary, and may be multiple for any one agent. Some have a local anaesthetic-like action, reducing cellular excitability through their effect on the sodium-dependent phase of depolarization. Others oppose the effect of catecholamines by decreasing excitability, conduction, and the ease with which ventricular fibrillation can begin. A third mechanism is by an effect on repolarization, lengthening the refractory period of cells. Drugs may also make the repolarization time of cardiac tissue more uniform across the heart; this has a stabilizing action. Finally, anti-arrhythmic drugs may oppose calcium-channel activity in cardiac cells. Calcium channels play an important part in the normal function of the sinoatrial and atrioventricular nodes, and appear central to the abnormal 'micro-re-entry' conduction that occurs in infarcted or severely ischaemic myocardium, leading to ventricular tachycardia or fibrillation.

These broad divisions of mechanism are reflected in the often-quoted Vaughan-Williams classification of anti-arrhythmic drugs (Table 8.2). This classification is based on a

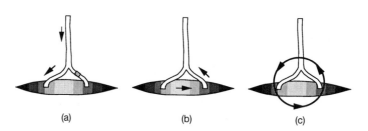

(a)　　　　　(b)　　　　　(c)

Fig. 8.4 ● A diagram to show micro re-entry in the terminal part of the Purkinje system and damaged myofibrils. (a) Forward passage of an impulse finds one limb of the Purkinje network blocked. (b) The impulse travels in the remaining limb, then slowly through the damaged muscle fibre until it can activate the hitherto refractory Purkinje fibre in a retrograde direction. (c) A re-entry circuit is then formed that can maintain a tachycardia.

Table 8.2 ● The Vaughan-Williams classification of anti-arrhythmic drugs

Mechanism	Examples
Class I: The 'local anaesthetic' agents	
All: oppose fast inward Na^+ current and reduce rise in action potential	
Ia: also prolong refractory period	Procainamide
	Disopyramide
Ib: do not extend refractory period	Lignocaine
	Mexiletine
Ic: also reduce conduction velocity	Flecainide
	Encainide
	Propafenone
Class II: The antisympathetic drugs	
Competitive beta blockade	All beta blockers
Non-competitive anti-adrenergic action	Bretylium
Class III: The 'antithyroid'drugs	
Prolongation of refractory period, but no effect on initial action potential	Amiodarone
	Sotalol
Class IV: The calcium-channel blockers	
Calcium-channel blockade	Verapamil
	Diltiazem

mechanism of cellular action rather than on either clinical effects or therapeutic usefulness; but it has remained a convenient framework for the discussion of anti-arrhythmic agents. The division between the Vaughan-Williams classes is by no means watertight, and the ability of a drug to raise the threshold for ventricular fibrillation (its so-called 'anti-fibrillatory action') is not specifically addressed by its place in this scheme.

Anti-arrhythmic drugs are used in two ways: to convert an abnormal rhythm to sinus rhythm (termination), or to prevent recurrence or worsening of an arrhythmia (prophylaxis). They are often effective—but are no panacea. Drugs inevitably have unwanted actions, often with unwelcome haemodynamic consequences. Dose titration for the desired effect is difficult, especially when the clinical state is highly unstable or where drug absorption is slow and unpredictable. The capacity of anti-arrhythmic drugs to cause arrhythmias—their so-called 'pro-arrhythmic effect'—is now well recognized, and may be responsible for their negligible or adverse influence on long-term mortality in patients with recurrent ventricular arrhythmias. The drawbacks of pharmacological agents have led to a renewed enthusiasm for electrical therapies to control tachycardia, as well as to maintain heart rate in profound bradycardia or asystole. Drugs remain of value, however, for prophylactic use and where electrical therapies are either unavailable or inadequate alone.

The following paragraphs describe additional anti-arrhythmic drugs likely to be used in life-threatening arrhythmias. They are listed according to the Vaughan-Williams classification.

Procainamide

Procainamide is a powerful anti-arrhythmic drug, with a concomitantly strong negative inotropic effect. It reduces the automaticity of ectopic pacemakers, slows interventricular conduction, and has a stronger antifibrillatory action than lignocaine. But it is rarely used to treat ventricular fibrillation, since adequate plasma levels are slow to be achieved even with intravenous administration.

For the treatment of ventricular tachycardia the recommended regimen is 50–100 mg boluses every 5 minutes, until the arrhythmia is suppressed, or blood pressure begins to fall, or a total dose of 500 mg has been given. Bolus doses are followed by an infusion beginning at 40 µg/kg/min (usually about 3 mg/min) to achieve a plasma level of 4–10 µg/ml. Doses should be reduced in renal impairment, and in any case should be as low as possible to achieve arrhythmia control. Careful monitoring of blood pressure, and a chest X-ray 4–6 hours after the initiation of therapy (to assess for pulmonary congestion) are also prudent to detect any significant cardiac failure. The ECG should be observed carefully for lengthening PR or QT intervals, widening of the QRS complex, or undue bradycardia.

Disopyramide

Disopyramide is a Class Ia drug with a wide spectrum of action. Excitability is reduced in atrial and ventricular muscle, and conduction is slowed in both myocardial cells and His Purkinje tissue. In addition—and this is peculiar to this drug—disopyramide has a marked atropinic (anticholinergic) effect that *increases* AV nodal conduction. For this reason disopyramide may have an adverse effect on the arrhythmias that depend on AV nodal refractoriness to limit ventricular rate (atrial flutter and fibrillation), and also on the arrhythmias of digitalis toxicity.

For the treatment of ventricular tachycardia and stubborn episodes of supraventricular tachycardia (p. 133) the dose is 2 mg/kg intravenously over 10–20 minutes to a maximum of 150 mg, repeated over 1 hour if necessary. No more than 300 mg should be given in the first hour. A maintenance infusion can be given subsequently at a rate of 20–30 mg per hour (400 µg/kg/hour), although the infusate should not be given or should be stopped when conversion to sinus rhythm occurs. Transfer to oral therapy is usual when the injection has been completed, by giving 200 mg disopyramide by mouth immediately, and then the same 8 hourly for the next 24 hours. Oral medication can be continued using the slow-release preparation if required. Dosage should be reduced in renal or hepatic failure.

The side-effects of disopyramide include the expected negative inotropic effect, which will combine with other anti-arrhythmic agents, including beta-blockers. In addition its atropinic effects may cause dry mouth, blurred vision, and urinary hesitancy, especially in the older male population. Side-effects usually disappear rapidly with a reduction in dose.

Flecainide

Characteristic of the newer Class Ic agents, flecainide is among the most effective drugs available for the treatment of ventricular and certain supraventricular arrhythmias. In addition to suppressing atrial and ventricular excitability, it markedly slows conduction throughout the heart. Even at therapeutic levels flecainide may prolong the PR interval and widen the QRS complex. Unlike many other anti-arrhythmic drugs, however, lengthening of the ST segment and the T wave does not occur.

Concerns have been expressed about flecainide's pro-arrhythmic effect. Although this property is shared by many anti-arrhythmic agents (Fig. 8.5), its ability to cause dangerous arrhythmias is more marked than that of many, in keeping with its more powerful anti-arrhythmic effect. It is advised primarily for the treatment of life-threatening ventricular arrhythmias, or for less sinister but symptomatic arrhythmias that cannot be controlled by other agents.

The dose in emergency situations is 2 mg/kg, to a maximum of 150 mg given over 30 minutes. An infusion can be continued if necessary at 1.5 mg/kg for the first hour, and then at 0.1–0.25 mg/kg per hour. This will usually achieve the required plasma level of 200–400 ng/ml. Dose reductions in the infusate are required in renal impairment, and a careful watch should be made for predictable side-effects: myocardial depression, bradycardia, or worsened ventricular arrhythmias.

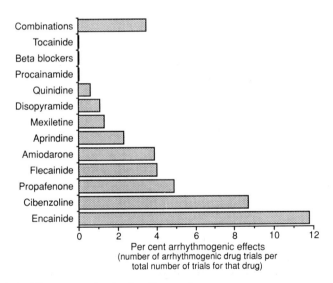

Fig. 8.5 ● The pro-arrhythmic effects of anti-arrhythmic agents. Data from a comparison of 1268 trials in 506 patients. Initial presentation in sustained VT (rather than non-sustained VT or VF) and poor systolic function make arrhythmogenesis more likely.

Beta-blockers

In Class II of the Vaughan-Williams classification, beta blockers have a modest anti-arrhythmic effect in competitively opposing cardiac β_1 receptors. Their stabilizing effect on cardiac rhythm may also gain from an opposition to β_2-mediated hypokalaemia. They are most effective for the control of recurrent ventricular tachycardia or fibrillation associated with ischaemic heart disease, or where the effect of circulating catecholamines is marked (thyrotoxicosis, recent withdrawal of beta blockers, or certain cardiomyopathies). They have no effect on the arrhythmia mechanisms that result from the stimulation of adrenergic α receptors.

Beta blockers have no place in the present protocols for the management of cardiac arrest; but their use should be considered early for recurrent VT associated with unstable angina or infarction. Failure of control by lignocaine, a resting tachycardia, mildly (but not severely) impaired left ventricular function, or hypertension are additional pointers to their use.

For non-urgent cases oral atenolol 50 mg twice a day is an appropriate starting regimen. If required more urgently, atenolol can be given intravenously in a dose of 5 mg over 5 minutes repeated 15 minutes later.

Where concern exists over left ventricular function, cautious introduction of metoprolol may be wise. This agent has a relatively short half-life, and can be given in initial doses as low as 12.5–25 mg three times a day. A newly available ultra-short-acting blocker, esmolol (Brevibloc), is proving useful to explore the effect of beta blockade on cardiovascular function in high-risk cases. Its action lasts only 5 to 10 minutes after a single bolus injection. If tolerated, a more prolonged infusion can be given, or a more familiar beta blocker can be used in its place.

Amiodarone

Amiodarone is the index—and virtually sole member—of the Class III anti-arrhythmic agents. It is a particularly effective drug.

Amiodarone prolongs action-potential duration and refractory period in atrial and ventricular muscle, with little or no effect on the initial phase of depolarization. It has an anti-fibrillatory action, but its effect on AV nodal and His–Purkinje conduction is weak. Its effect on ventricular muscle commends its use in refractory or recurrent ventricular arrhythmias, particularly as its adverse effect on myocardial contractility is more benign than that of almost all other effective anti-arrhythmic drugs. A powerful action on atrial muscle and atrioventricular bypass tracts also makes it effective in supraventricular tachycardias. It has a unique success in suppressing paroxysmal atrial arrhythmias (atrial fibrillation, atrial flutter and atrial ectopic tachycardia).

For the control of life-threatening arrhythmias, intravenous amiodarone is indicated in a dose of 900 mg infused in 5 per cent dextrose over 90 minutes. The infusion rate can be faster if clinical needs dictate, but in all cases the drug should be given as centrally as possible; thrombophlebitis is almost universal if it is given into a peripheral vein.

For less urgent cases, but where parenteral therapy is required, a dose of 300 mg infused over 30–60 minutes three times a day is appropriate.

Where the drug can be given orally, a loading regimen of 200 mg three times a day for one week, and then 200 mg twice a day as maintenance seems appropriate. For the long-term treatment of supraventricular tachycardias a maintenance dose of 200 mg daily may be sufficient, particularly in the elderly.

The unique spectrum and efficacy of amiodarone is offset by an impressive list of potential side-effects. In the heart it has a pro-arrhythmic and a mildly negative inotropic effect. The commonest non-cardiac side-effect is the corneal deposition of lipofucsin. This occurs with therapeutic amiodarone levels in more than 90 per cent of patients, but is rarely troublesome, and hardly ever requires discontinuation of therapy. Beware, too, of potential interactions with digoxin and with warfarin, of important disorders of thyroid function (for which the patient should be screened regularly), and of the development of pulmonary fibrosis.

Sotalol

Sotalol is a beta blocker, but with additional anti-arrhythmic properties beyond those attributable to beta blockade alone.

The usual preparation is a racemic mixture; but the two optical isomers have different anti-arrhythmic actions. The *l*-form possesses non-cardioselective beta blocking effects; and the *d*-form is almost devoid of beta blocking activity, but has a Class III effect. The racaemic mixture is therefore useful as prophylactic treatment for recurrent arrhythmias where a Class III action could be of help (atrial arrhythmias or supraventricular tachycardias). The use of *d*-sotalol alone appears, however, to add no specific clinical advantage to the use of the racemic compound.

Calcium-channel blocking agents

Calcium-channel blocking drugs offer a spectrum of effect that varies with the individual agent. Activity is spread between peripheral vascular smooth muscle, coronary vascular smooth muscle, the myocardium, and the conducting system. The most powerful anti-arrhythmic calcium-channel blocker is verapamil. It has a suppressant action on pacemaker tissue in the sinoatrial and atrioventricular nodes, and is therefore specially useful in tachycardias that involve these structures.

Verapamil is commonly used intravenously for the conversion of supraventricular tachycardias. A slow intravenous injection of no more than 10 mg should be given for this indication, and will produce a peak therapeutic effect within 3 to 5 minutes. Caution needs to be exercised, because a combined effect with beta blockers can have serious consequences. Verapamil given to patients taking a beta blocker can produce a profoundly negative chronotropic and inotropic effect, and fatalities have been reported. Verapamil will safely enhance the AV nodal suppressant effect of digoxin, and no undue myocardial depression is threatened by this combination.

Other agents

Magnesium

Magnesium occupies a position of growing popularity as an adjunct to arrhythmic therapy. Intracellular magnesium depletion commonly accompanies chronic diuretic therapy, and is as arryhthmogenic as a low potassium state. Not all 'potassium-retaining' diuretics exert a similar salutory effect on magnesium.

By its effect on slow sodium channels, magnesium therapy may exert a specific anti-arrhythmic effect, in addition to correcting intracellular electrolyte imbalance. It also has the overwhelming advantage of leaving ventricular function unsuppressed. The dose is 50 ml of a 50 per cent solution infused over 30 minutes. This may be repeated once or even twice, and is frequently worth using in addition to all other therapy when ventricular arrhythmias are resistant to conventional therapy or patients have received diuretics.

Digoxin

It is difficult to find a natural 'home' for digoxin in a classification of anti-arrhythmic drugs! Its important action is slowing AV nodal conduction for supraventricular tachycardias (particularly atrial fibrillation) is well known, and it is likely also to have at least a transient positive inotropic effect in the failing myocardium. It carries an additional advantage that any increase in cardiac contractility that results from its use appears to occur with little increase in oxygen demand.

Theoretically, the cardiac glycosides decrease the threshold for ventricular fibrillation, particularly in the face of myocardial ischaemia, infarction, hypokalaemia, and hypomagnesaemia. In practice, however, the prudent use of digoxin for rapid atrial arrhythmias even in unstable angina or acute myocardial infarction appears safe, provided that concomitant attention is paid to potassium and magnesium replacement. The dose schedules are outlined in Chapter 7, p. 140.

Calcium

Calcium ions increase the force of contraction of the heart, and are essential for the coupling between depolarization (excitation) and mechanical shortening of myocardial cells. They have a variable effect on peripheral resistance, although they are present in significant quantities in the myocytes of arteriolar smooth muscle.

No data demonstrate a beneficial effect of calcium salts given therapeutically during resuscitation. Theoretically, they can add to myocardial damage following myocardial infarction, and can adversely affect the neurological outcome of patients after cardiac arrest. Their use is permissible for acute hypocalcaemia, hyperkalaemia, or calcium-channel blocker toxicity. The dose is 10 ml of 10 per cent solution of calcium chloride, which contains 13.6 mEq of calcium. It cannot be mixed with sodium bicarbonate, and should be used with caution in patients on digitalis.

Adenosine

Adenosine, although an indigenous compound throughout the body, has profound, usable, though very short-lived, electrophysiological actions when administered intravenously. Its chief effect is in depressing AV nodal conduction with a half-life of 2–10 seconds. With intravenous use, it will often convert a paroxysmal supraventricular tachycardia to sinus rhythm, particularly in the common situation where AV nodal re-entry is the underlying mechanism. It can also aid the diagnosis of a broad complex tachycardia where the rhythm (ventricular tachycardia versus supraventricular tachycardia with aberrant conduction) is unclear.

Adenosine is given by rapid intravenous bolus injection over 2 seconds followed by a saline flush. Use 3 mg initially and, if required a second dose of 6 mg and a third dose of 12 mg at 1 to 2 minute intervals. Care should be taken with asthmatic patients since adenosine is a bronchoconstrictor. Other side-effects include flushing and headache, although adenosine's short half-life limits the duration of any unwanted effect.

Further reading

1. Aronson, J. K. (1985). Cardiac arrhythmias: theory and practice. *British Medical Journal*, **290**, 487–8.
2. Brown, C. G. and Werman, H. A. (1990). Adrenergic antagonists during cardiopulmonary resuscitation. *Resuscitation*, **19**, 1–16.
3. Capparelli, E. V., Chow, M. S. S., Kluger, J. and Felman, A. (1989). Differences in systemic and myocardial blood acid–base status during cardiopulmonary resuscitation. *Critical Care Medicine*, **17**, 442–6.

4. Dorian, P., Fain, E. S., Davy, J. M. and Winkle, R. A. (1986). Lidocaine causes a reversible, concentration-dependent increase in defibrillation energy requirements. *Journal of the American College of Cardiology*, **8**, 327–32.
5. Grundler, W., Weil, M. H. and Rackow, E. C. (1986). Arteriovenous carbon dioxide and pH gradients during cardiac arrest. *Circulation*, **74**, 1071–4.
6. Kerber, R. E. and Sarnot, W. (1979). Factors influencing the success of ventricular defibrillation in man. *Circulation*, **60**, 226–30.
7. MacMahon, S., Collins, R., Peto, R., Koster, R. W. and Yusuf, S. (1988). Effects of prophylactic lidocaine in suspected acute myocardial infarction: an overview of results from the randomized controlled trials. *Journal of the American Medical Association*, **260**, 1910–16.
8. Olson, D. W., Thompson, B. M., Darin, J. C. and Milbrath, M. H. (1984). A randomized comparison study of bretylium tosylate and lidocaine in resuscitation of patients from out-of-hospital ventricular fibrillation in a paramedic system. *Annals of Emergency Medicine*, **13**, 807–10.
9. Opie, L. H. (1991). *Drugs for the heart*, (3rd edn). W. B. Saunders, Philadelphia.
10. Ornato, J. P., Gonzalez, E. R., Starke, H., Morkunas, A., Coyne, M. R. and Beck, C. L. (1985). Incidence and causes of hypokalaemia associated with cardiac resuscitation. *American Journal of Emergency Medicine*, **3**, 503–6.
11. Paradis, N. A. and Koscove, E. M. (1990). Epinephrine in cardiac arrest, a critical review. *Annals of Emergency Medicine*, **19**, 1288–301.
12. Rankin, A. C., Roe, A. P. and Cobbe, S. M. (1987). Misuse of intravenous verapamil in patients with ventricular tachycardia. *Lancet*, **ii**, 472–4.
13. Rice, V. (1987). Acid–base derangements in the patient with cardiac arrest. *Focus on Critical Care*, **14**, 56–61.
14. Sanders, A. B., Otto, C. W., Kern, K. B., Rogers, J. N., Perrault, P. and Ewy, G. A. (1988). Acid–base balance in a canine model of cardiac arrest. *Annals of Emergency Medicine*, **17**, 667–71.
15. Schmitz, B., Fischer, M., Bockhurst, K., Hoehn-Berlage, M. and Hossmannm, K-A. (1995). Resuscitation from cardiac arrest in cats: influence of epinephrine dosage on brain recovery. *Resuscitation*, **30**, 251–62.
16. Stanton, M. S., Prystowski, E. N., Fineberg, N. S., Miles, W. M., Zipes, D. P. and Heger, J. J. (1989). Arrhythmogenic effect of antiarrhythmic drugs: A study of 506 patients treated for ventric-

ular tachycardia or fibrillation. *Journal of the American College of Cardiology*, **14**, 209–15.

17. Van Planta, M., Weil, M. H., Gazmuri, R. J., Bisera, J. and Rackow, E. C. (1989). Myocardial acidosis with CO_2 production during cardiac arrest and resuscitation. *Circulation*, **80**, 684–92.

18. Weil, M. H., Ring, C. E., Michaels, S. and Rackow, E. C. (1985). Acid–base determinants of survival after cardiopulmonary resuscitation. *Critical Care Medicine*, **13**, 88–92.

19. Woodhouse, S. P., Cox, S., Boyd, P., Case, C. and Weber, M. (1995). High dose and standard dose adrenaline do not alter survival, compared with placebo, in cardiac arrest. *Resuscitation*, **30**, 243–9.

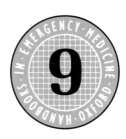

CHAPTER 9

Paediatric resuscitation

Key points in paediatric resuscitation

1 Hypoxia is the most common cause of cardiac arrest in children.

2 Opening the airway is the first and most important point of the resuscitation sequence in infants. Thus, it is essential to follow the classic **A**irway, **B**reathing, **C**irculation sequence.

3 Airway obstruction may occur as a result of inhalation of a foreign body. Clear the airway with back blows. Only use abdominal thrusts in older children.

4 Airway obstruction occurring as a result of airway infection requires urgent expert care.

5 Infants are nasal breathers. Cover the mouth and nose to perform expired air respiration.

6 Check the circulation by palpating the brachial pulse.

7 In infants, perform chest compression one finger's-breadth below the inter-nipple line, at a rate of 100 compressions per minute to a depth of 1.0–1.5 cm.

8 Advanced paediatric cardiac life support requires formal training in techniques of airway management, intravenous cannulation, and intraosseous infusion.

9 Although the paediatric algorithms for advanced resuscitation closely resemble those for adults, it is essential not to treat infants as small adults, and to calculate formally the required drug dosage by extrapolating from age, weight, or length.

Introduction

Paediatric resuscitation follows the same essential principles as adult resuscitation. The difference is that paediatric resuscitation events occur over a wide range of size and weight, varying from the small baby, at 2.5 kg, to the average teenager, at 70 kg. With this wide range, it is obvious that the paediatric resuscitator must have knowledge of and confidence in the methods appropriate to the size of child.

This chapter will deal mainly with the small infant weighing between 5 and 10 kg. Patients at the other end of the range can be dealt with as small adults. It will not deal with resuscitation of the newborn, as this is a specialist, planned recovery event occurring in the delivery room. Suggested further reading on resuscitation of the newborn is given at the end of the chapter.

In the United Kingdom in 1987, 6272 infants died aged under one year, of whom 3448 (55 per cent) died in the first month. During the same period 11.3 per cent of deaths in children aged 28 days to 14 years were due to accidental causes; in the age group 5–14 years, 32 per cent of deaths were recorded as accidental. Thus, although paediatric resuscitation is often reported as being uncommon, there are a substantial number of paediatric resuscitation events where effective treatment schedules could possibly have improved the eventual outcome.

Aetiology of paediatric cardiac arrest

The primary aetiology of cardiac arrest in infants and children is different from that in adults. Hypoxia is the most common cause, and a primary cardiac event is rarely seen. Other notable causes are sudden infant death syndrome, loss of blood or body fluids resulting in circulatory hypovolaemia, congenital heart disease, and septicaemia. Despite differences in aetiology, the aims of resuscitation are the same as those in any other resuscitation event. Providing an airway, establishing breathing, and restoring the circulation are tasks which, when properly carried out, can improve prognosis and may lead to survival. Unfortunately, paediatric resuscitation is approached with much emotion, apprehension, and uncertainty. Treatment must commence immediately to be effective; delays in recognizing or treating a cardiac arrest or therapeutic mistakes may seriously affect the outcome.

Basic cardiac life support

Importance of the ABC approach

In resuscitation in infants and children, follow the sequence:
Airway
Breathing
Circulation
This is even more appropriate than usual in this resuscitation group, as the commonest cause of collapse is hypoxia which may be remedied by the simple technique of airway control, thus preventing the further progression of the event.

Airway

Open the airway by tilting the head and supporting the lower-jaw (Fig. 9.1). Jaw-support is an essential part of this manoeuvre, as it will displace the relatively large infant tongue forward from the posterior pharyngeal wall. Care must be taken not to press on the soft tissues behind the chin, as this will force the tongue into the airway and cause obstruction. Over-extension of the head on the neck must also be avoided,

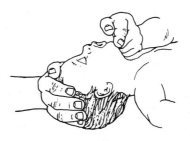

Fig. 9.1 ● Open the airway.

as this may kink the airway. A small support placed behind the shoulders may aid neck extension and stabilize the position. The optimal position for head-tilt and jaw-support varies from child to child, and even in experienced hands it is a matter of trying various positions and choosing the best result. The selected position must be frequently reassessed, and the rescuer must be flexible enough in his technique to allow for readjustment.

Infants are obligatory nose-breathers. Careful clearing of the nasal passages by suction, and the removal of iatrogenic obstructions, such as nasogastric tubes, will aid the child's return to spontaneous respiration.

Airway obstruction

Inhalation of food, vomit, or a foreign body into the airway is not uncommon in children. In the United States one child dies every five days from asphyxiation due to the inhalation of food. Although education about prevention will reduce this toll, the immediate management of an obstructed airway should be public knowledge.

Careful removal of any visible foreign body is essential to avoid making the situation worse. Techniques such as blind finger-probing, or finger-sweeps, may result in further impaction of the object, or may traumatize the upper airway, causing oedema and haemorrhage. If simple removal is not effective then the child must be inverted, and four back-blows applied to the middle of the back (Figs 9.2 and 9.3).

This procedure has a dual effect. The vibration from the back-blow may loosen the object from the impacted position. Secondly, each back-blow causes a rapid chest compression, resulting in increased intrathoracic pressure and a miniature 'cough'. Formal abdominal thrusts can be applied to children over the age of 5 years. Following the back-slaps the child's airway should be carefully investigated for the displaced foreign body.

Infection of the upper airway, often called croup, but including simple laryngitis, acute laryngotracheobronchitis, and epiglottitis, can also cause airway obstruction. A high index of suspicion, prompt recognition, correct diagnosis, and

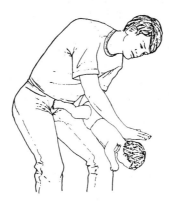

Fig. 9.2 ● Back-blows for an obstructed airway (infant).

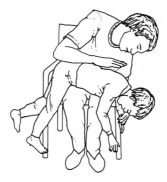

Fig. 9.3 ● Back-blows for an obstructed airway (child).

proper management can avert a crisis. In the initial stages the child may prefer to sit up, and even to lean forward, to allow the saliva to dribble away. Humidification of the room air is also helpful. Early transport, with adequate supervision and monitoring, to a paediatric intensive care unit is recommended, as further active intervention on site, no matter how well intentioned, could have disastrous consequences. In hospital, distress should be avoided and careful monitoring should be continued. Examination of the oropharynx, laryn-goscopy, and intubation of the trachea should only be attempted in the operating theatre by an experienced anaes-thetist in the presence of an ENT surgeon.

Breathing

Spontaneous respiratory efforts can be checked for by

– looking for smooth and symmetrical chest-wall movement;
– *listening* for breath sounds; and
– *feeling* for air movement over the mouth.

Irregular chest wall movements, intercostal recession, see-saw movements of the chest and abdomen, flaring of the nostrils, and tracheal tug all indicate increased work in breathing and possible airway obstruction. This can often be simply dealt with by repositioning the airway.

If spontaneous respiratory efforts are absent then artificial ventilation must commence immediately. This is performed as expired air respiration. In the infant, the mouth and nose of the infant are covered with the rescuer's mouth (Fig. 9.4). Blow into the mouth and nose until the infant's chest begins to rise. At this point stop blowing and allow the infant to breath out. In the older child the same procedure is followed, except that only the mouth of the child is covered, the nose being occluded by pinching the nostrils shut.

Give *two breaths*. If one stops blowing when the chest starts to move, over-inflation of the lungs does not occur. Over-infla-

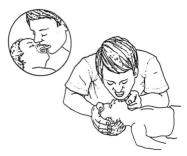

Fig. 9.4 ● Mouth-to-mouth and nose expired air respiration.

tion or the use of high airway pressures should be avoided, as they may cause gastric distension and vomiting.

Circulation

The circulation is usually checked by feeling for the carotid pulse in the neck. Infants, however have relatively short, fat necks, and feeling for the brachial pulse on the inner aspect of the upper arm is more accurate (Fig. 9.5). Time must be taken in assessing the pulse, especially if there is a bradycardia or an abnormal rhythm. Bradycardias are a common accompaniment to hypoxic episodes in children. A bradycardia in an infant or a small child is any pulse rate below 80 beats per minute.

If no pulse is felt, or if there is a profound bradycardia, then external chest compressions must be commenced to maintain the circulation. The heart lies under the lower third of the sternum, and thus chest compressions should be applied to the junction of the lower and middle thirds of the sternum (Fig. 9.6). In the small infant chest compressions are carried out at a position one finger's-breadth below the inter-nipple line, or the same distance above the xiphisternum. Using the tips of two fingers compress 1.0–1.5 cm at a rate of 100 per minute, alternating five compressions with one breath. In the older child over the age of five years, the position moves to two finger's-breadths above the xiphisternum. Use the heel of one or both hands, compressing 2–3 cm at a rate of 100 per minute, alternating 15 compressions with 2 breaths. The precision of the rate, depth, and method of compression is not of vital importance. Adaptability of technique must be foremost

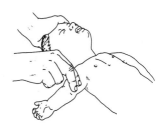

Fig. 9.5 ● Brachial pulse check.

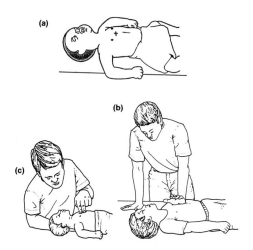

Fig. 9.6 ● (a) Chest compression position. (b) Chest compression in infants. (c) Chest compression in children.

in the resuscitator's mind. It is all important to produce the best circulation of oxygenated blood, whatever the method selected.

Basic life support must be continued until advanced cardiac life support is started. Basic life support effectively 'buys time'; but it is only the advanced life support drugs and equipment which have the potential of providing a successful recovery.

Advanced cardiac life support

Importance of training and experience

To be truly effective the use of equipment in advanced cardiac life support requires training and experience. This is especially so in paediatric resuscitation, as there is a wide range of equipment available to match the various sizes of children encountered.

Airway

Guedel airway The simplest airway device is the Guedel airway. Even at this simple level there is a range of choice for sizes, from 000 to 4. If too small an airway is selected then it will not overcome the obstruction of the tongue, and may force the tongue to the back of the pharynx. Too large an airway may damage the posterior pharyngeal wall as the airway is rotated into position. In the older child the airway is best inserted into the mouth upside-down, and then rotated 180 degrees into the correct position as the tip of the airway reaches the roof of the mouth. This method is not so appropriate in small children. The correct size should position comfortably in the mouth, with the teeth or alveolar ridges resting on the bite-block. In many children, therefore, a Guedel airway may only complicate airway management. If this is found to be the case it should be omitted, and only the careful use of head, neck, and jaw positions should be used to control the airway.

Nasal airway If the pharyngeal reflexes are present or if there is difficulty in positioning an oral airway, then a nasal airway can be used. An uncuffed tracheal tube of suitable size, cut to a short length, is the simplest form of nasal airway. A nasal airway must be carefully secured to prevent it disappearing into the nares.

Tracheal airway Tracheal intubation is the only way of providing a guaranteed airway. Intubation is a skill only acquired through repeated training and practice. A full range of sizes and lengths of tracheal tubes must be available. The correct size is selected by using the age of the child in reference to a simple chart (Fig. 9.8) or by using the formula: (age in years ÷ 4) + 4 = internal diameter of the tracheal tube in millimetres (Box 9.1, Table 9.1). The tracheal tube must also be cut to the

---

Box 9.1 • Determining the correct tracheal tube size for infants

$$\text{Tracheal tube size (internal diameter in mm)} = \frac{\text{Age in years}}{4} = 4$$

Table 9.1 ● Table of tracheal tube sizes by age in years

Age (years)	Endotracheal tube internal diameter (mm)	Length (cm)		Suction catheter (FG)
		Oral	Nasal	
Premature	2.5–3.0	11	13.5	6
Newborn	3.5	12	14	8
1	4.0	13	15	8
2	4.5	14	16	8
4	5.0	15	17	10
6	5.5	17	19	10
8	6.0	19	21	10
10	6.5	20	22	10
12	7.0	21	22	10
14	7.5	22	23	10
16	8.0	23	24	12

appropriate length (see Fig. 9.8) to prevent intubation of the left or right main bronchus.

Intubation in small children (under 8 years) is best achieved using an uncuffed tracheal tube and a straight blade laryngoscope. In children over the age of 8 years (6 mm tracheal tube size) a cuffed tracheal tube and a curved blade laryngoscope can be used. In an emergency, the flat end of a curved adult laryngoscope blade can be carefully used if a straight laryngoscope blade is not available. When the trachea has been intubated the tube must be secured firmly in a position to prevent accidental movement or inadvertent extubation. The position of the tip of the tube must be checked by auscultation of the chest to ensure that the right or left main bronchi have not been entered inadvertently, resulting in the ventilation of only one lung. If one-lung ventilation is diagnosed then the tracheal tube should be withdrawn slowly until bilateral and equal air entry is auscultated.

A wide range of tracheal tube connectors is available. The 15 mm British Standard connector will fit directly on to the self-inflating resuscitation bag without the need for any intermediate connector, and is recommended for its simplicity. If any other connector is used then it is essential that an appropriate adaptor for the connector is available. The appropriate

size of suction catheter must also be provided together with a
rigid Yankauer suction catheter to maintain a clear upper airway (see Fig. 6.7, p. 104). Having established the airway, it is
essential to recheck constantly that the airway is being properly maintained, and has not become occluded by an anatomical obstruction, by kinking, or by airway secretions.

Breathing

It is essential to increase the oxygen concentration of the
inspired air of the collapsed child as early as possible in the
resuscitation sequence. Supplemental oxygen via a face mask,
nasal cannulae, or an oxygen tent may provide an initial
solution; but if the child is not breathing, then a method of
artificial ventilation must be used.

Artificial ventilation This is performed by using a self-inflating resuscitation bag, valve, and mask. There are three sizes of
resuscitation bag (Table 9.2). The two smaller bags have a
pressure-limited valve preset to 45 cm of water, to prevent
over-pressurization of a child's lungs during inflation. This
valve can be overridden in cases where a high airway resistance or a decreased lung compliance is diagnosed and adequate ventilation is not being achieved at airway inflation
pressures below 45 cm of water.

The simplicity of the bag–valve–mask system may lead to
an exaggerated belief in its effectiveness. Many studies have
shown the low tidal volumes achieved when using this system, especially when in inexperienced hands. A circular-
shaped mask is easier to use than the conventional paediatric
Rendell–Baker-shaped mask. A mask made of clear plastic is
recommended, regardless of its shape, so that the skin colour
of the child can be assessed easily, together with the presence
or absence of secretions, without the need to remove the mask

Table 9.2 ● Resuscitation bag volumes

Age and weight	Bag volume (ml)	Tidal volume (ml)
<2 years (<7kg)	240	205
2–10 years (7–30 kg)	500	350
>10 years (>30 kg)	1600	1000

from the face. Ventilation can always be assessed as effective if the simple rule is followed that the chest must be seen to move with each ventilation. Practice improves performance; but if ventilation fails then there must be a return to the expired air method. The 22 mm connector of the resuscitation bag fits directly to the 15 mm tracheal tube connector. Supplemental oxygen can be added to the inspiratory port of the resuscitation bag, and boosted to high oxygen percentages by the use of an inspiratory gas reservoir bag.

Automatic ventilators are not recommended for use with children. This is especially true with pressure-cycled ventilators, as these will be pre-triggered by the chest compression procedures themselves. Paediatric ventilation requires constant monitoring and repeated evaluation to ensure that it is adequate and safe.

Circulation

Importance of repeated measurement of vital signs Circulation must be assessed by an electrocardiogram, together with repeated pulse and blood pressure measurements. Bradycardias in children are as detrimental as asystole. In infants and babies a pulse rate below 60 beats per minute must be considered a profound bradycardia.

The management of the child's circulation requires both physiological and pharmacological intervention. Blood pressure measurements taken by an indirect method, a blood pressure cuff, depend on the width of the cuff in relation to the size of the child's arm. A single measurement on its own is of little use. Multiple measurements, indicating a physiological change, are of more value provided the same equipment is used each time.

Children tolerate hypovolaemia poorly, but will maintain their blood pressure by raising their heart rate until a loss of at least 25 per cent of circulating blood volume has occurred. Hypervolaemia can also cause problems, and may present as a bradycardia associated with a low or normal blood pressure.

Intravenous access Circulatory management requires the establishment of intravenous access at the earliest opportunity. This is one of the major problems in paediatric resuscitation. The choice of route and of cannula is one of personal preference and experience; but it must always be remembered that access is of primary importance, and adequate resuscitation can be commenced even through a cannula of a size as small as 24 SWG.

Central venous access This is preferable for drug administration to peripheral access, and there are a number of routes to choose from:

• internal jugular vein;
• external jugular vein;
• subclavian vein; and
• femoral vein.

Of these four routes, the external jugular vein is usually very prominent during arrest situations, and provides simple visible access. The internal jugular route requires a highly specialized technique, and the subclavian route runs the risk of causing a pneumothorax or haemothorax. The femoral route may be acceptable for short-term access, but is often regarded as a 'dirty venous access'. Drugs administered from a subdiaphragmatic route take longer to act and are less effective.

Peripheral venous access If central venous access fails then peripheral access is the next best choice. Many favour the vein found in the antecubital fossa. It suffers from the disadvantage that all drugs must be flushed centrally, and therefore repeated drug administration could easily result in inadvertent fluid overload.

Other routes (tracheal, intraosseous, intracardiac Other routes that may be considered are:

Tracheal drug administration Adrenaline, atropine, and lignocaine can be given down the tracheal tube for absorption by the pulmonary vascular bed. Drugs are best given through a long cannula passed to the distal end of the tracheal tube; and the lungs are hyperventilated for 5 to 7 breaths following administration. Double the normal intravenous dose of drug is recommended when using the tracheal route.

Intraosseous drug and fluid administration An intraosseous infusion needle can be inserted 1 cm below the tibial plateau on the anterior surface of the tibia. Drugs and fluids can be administered by this route, and absorption into the circulation is as rapid as in intravenous infusion. All administrations are best given by pressure infusion. The main contraindication is a proximal long-bone fracture.

Intracardiac drug administration This route is not recommended, because not only does it necessitate stopping cardiac compression, but it has been shown that the majority of attempted intracardiac injections miss the heart. It should also be remembered that there is a high risk of myocardial laceration or coronary vessel damage with a blind percutaneous approach.

Whichever route is used, a careful record must be kept of all drugs and fluids administered. A running tally of the overall fluid load administered must be maintained, keeping a watch for potential circulatory overload.

Management of arrhythmias

There are designated protocols for the three major rhythms associated with cardiac arrest. These are for:

- ventricular fibrillation (VF);
- asystole; and
- electromechanical dissociation (EMD).

Ventricular fibrillation

Ventricular fibrillation (VF) is not seen as commonly in children as in adults, and is usually secondary to another cardiac insult. It is characterized as electromechanical anarchy, with an electrocardiographic trace like that shown above.

The management of VF is defibrillation (Fig. 9.7): the passage of an electric current across the myocardium. If the arrest is witnessed then an initial precordial thump can be administered. In children a first defibrillation shock is given at 2 joules per kilogram of body weight (see Fig. 9.8). The defibrillator paddles are selected according to the size of the child. The standard defibrillation position is used. However, it may be easier to apply the paddles in the anterior-posterior position, across the chest wall of the infant. Paddle-size selection is made by choosing the largest size of paddle which provides the best contact with the chest wall. Certain defibrillators will

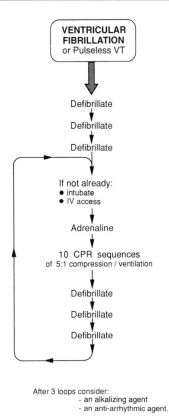

**VENTRICULAR
FIBRILLATION**
or Pulseless VT

Defibrillate

Defibrillate

Defibrillate

If not already:
● intubate
● IV access

Adrenaline

10 CPR sequences
of 5:1 compression / ventilation

Defibrillate

Defibrillate

Defibrillate

After 3 loops consider:
- an alkalizing agent
- an anti-arrhythmic agent.

Fig. 9.7 ● Flowchart for the management of ventricular fibrillation (VF). (Dosages and energies are provided in Fig. 9.8).

only charge to preset levels (20, 50, 100, 200, or 360 J), while others have a preset maximum dose of 100 J when paediatric paddles are connected. It may therefore be necessary to approximate the calculated energy dose to the nearest level achievable through the machine. Following the initial 2 shocks at 2 joules per kilogram, further shocks of 4 joules per kilogram are given if VF persists.

After the third defibrillation, *adrenaline* is given, either intravenously at 10 μg/kg (0.1 ml/kg of 1 in 10 000 solution) or via the tracheal tube (20 μg/kg). This is the front-line drug in resuscitation, and acts primarily through its α adrenergic

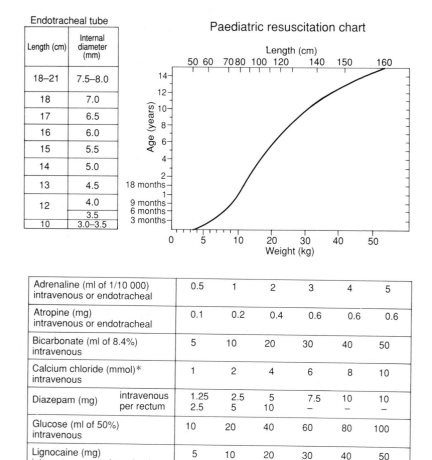

Endotracheal tube

Length (cm)	Internal diameter (mm)
18–21	7.5–8.0
18	7.0
17	6.5
16	6.0
15	5.5
14	5.0
13	4.5
12	4.0
	3.5
10	3.0–3.5

Paediatric resuscitation chart

Adrenaline (ml of 1/10 000) intravenous or endotracheal	0.5	1	2	3	4	5
Atropine (mg) intravenous or endotracheal	0.1	0.2	0.4	0.6	0.6	0.6
Bicarbonate (ml of 8.4%) intravenous	5	10	20	30	40	50
Calcium chloride (mmol)* intravenous	1	2	4	6	8	10
Diazepam (mg) intravenous	1.25	2.5	5	7.5	10	10
Diazepam (mg) per rectum	2.5	5	10	–	–	–
Glucose (ml of 50%) intravenous	10	20	40	60	80	100
Lignocaine (mg) intravenous or endotracheal	5	10	20	30	40	50
Salbutamol (micrograms) intravenous	25	50	100	150	200	250
Initial DC deflbrillation (J)	10	20	40	60	80	100
Initial fluid infusion in hypovolaemic shock (ml)	50	100	200	300	400	500

* One millilitre calcium chloride 1 mmol/ml ≡ 1.5 ml calcium chloride 10% ≡ 4.5 ml calcium gluconate 10%

Fig. 9.8 ● Paediatric resuscitation chart.

receptors, causing a rise in systemic vascular resistance. This increases the end-diastolic filling pressure and improves coronary perfusion. Adrenaline's α activity also 'stiffens' the major vessels carrying blood away from the heart, preventing their collapse, and thus increasing the effectiveness of chest compressions. The β adrenergic effects of adrenaline directly increase the inotropic and chronotropic activity of the myocardium.

Basic life support should follow the administration of adrenaline for 10 CPR sequences of 5 compressions to 1 ventilation. Further defibrillation attempts are made each at the higher energy (4 joules per kilogram) and further doses of adrenaline should be used if VF persists. In addition, a change in defibrillator paddle positions, the use of a different defibrillator, or the administration of anti-arrythmic drugs (e.g. lignocaine at 1 mg/kg bretylium at 4 mg/kg) may be considered.

Asystole

Asystolic or severe bradycardic cardiac arrests are seen most often in children. The most common cause is hypoxia, and therefore all treatment regimens must be aimed at correcting hypoxia by establishing an airway and effective ventilation with oxygen.

The management of asystole (Fig. 9.9): following attachment of the electrocardiograph, if ventricular fibrillation cannot be excluded, then the defibrillation schedule must be commenced. If the diagnosis of asystole is confirmed then adrenaline 10 µg/kg (0.1 ml/kg of a 1 in 10 000 solution) should be given either intravenously or via the tracheal tube. Following a period basic life support atropine 0.02 mg/kg (minimum 0.1 mg) should be administered via the same route if asystole persists. Atropine is a parasympathetic-blocking drug. It will directly inhibit the action of the vagus nerve on the heart, although its benefit in asystolic cardiac arrest is debatable. Administration of atropine has been known to cause VF where severe hypoxia exists.

External cardiac pacing may be considered in cases where P waves are seen on the ECG. Unfortunately, the results of external cardiac pacing have not been encouraging. This may be because it is commenced late in the resuscitation sequence,

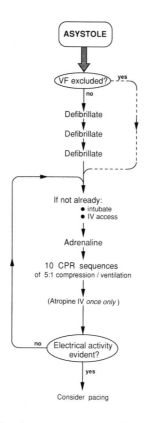

Fig. 9.9 ● Flowchart for the management of apparent asystole. (Dosages and energies are provided in Fig. 9.8).

when permanent damage to the myocardium has already occurred.

Electromechanical dissociation

The occurrence of a QRS complex on the ECG without a palpable pulse may be the result of trauma, hypovolaemia, pneumothorax, cardiac tamponade, or pulmonary embolism.

The management of EMD (Fig. 9.10): although urgent efforts should be made to correct the diagnosed condition, adrenaline 10 µg/kg (0.1 ml/kg of a 1 in 10 000 solution) will aid in sup-

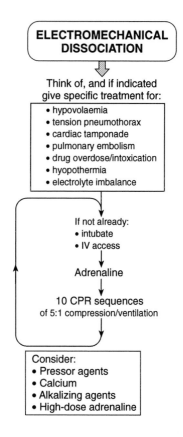

ELECTROMECHANICAL DISSOCIATION

Think of, and if indicated give specific treatment for:
- hypovolaemia
- tension pneumothorax
- cardiac tamponade
- pulmonary embolism
- drug overdose/intoxication
- hyopothermia
- electrolyte imbalance

If not already:
- intubate
- IV access

Adrenaline

10 CPR sequences
of 5:1 compression/ventilation

Consider:
- Pressor agents
- Calcium
- Alkalizing agents
- High-dose adrenaline

Fig. 9.10 ● Flowchart for the management of electromechanical dissociation (EMD). Dosages are provided in Fig. 9.8).

porting the circulation until other therapeutic corrections have been made.

EMD may also be seen in hypocalcaemia/hyperkalaemia or calcium-antagonist drug overdose. In these situations, calcium chloride 5–10 mg/kg (0.25 ml/kg of a 10 per cent solution) should be given intravenously into a central vein. Alternatively, 30 mg/kg of calcium gluconate can be given via a peripheral vein.

Prolonged resuscitation

Use of sodium bicarbonate Resuscitation should be a continuous process, with minimal interruption of basic life support. Acidosis may occur during a prolonged resuscitation, but can be kept within acceptable levels by effective ventilation and efficient chest compressions. Correction of acidosis in children after blood-gas analysis should only be attempted by administering sodium bicarbonate intravenously in a direct therapeutic titration to the formula:

$$\text{Body weight} \times 0.6 \times \text{base deficit} = \text{mmol of } HCO_3.$$

In the absence of blood-gas analysis an empirical dose of 0.5–1.0 mmol/kg sodium bicarbonate can be given in prolonged resuscitation attempts. Although it may be physiologically desirable to correct the acid–base balance it is more important not to make the child alkalotic from bicarbonate overdose. Sodium bicarbonate must never be given unless effective ventilation has been established. The side-effects of administering such an hypernatraemic and hyperosmolar solution must be balanced against its dubious beneficial effects.

Other useful drugs Dopamine in low dosage (1–5 μg/kg/min) will improve cardiac output and renal blood flow. In high doses (10–12 μg/kg/min) α adrenergic effects predominate, causing a systemic vasoconstriction. A rapid dose calculation can be made by adding 3 × body weight in mg of dopamine to 50 ml of 5 per cent dextrose and infusing the mixture in ml/hour equivalent to the does in μg/kg/min required.

Dextrose Hypoglycaemia is a well-documented cause of collapse in small infants, as they have low levels of stored glycogen. This is especially so in the chronically sick child. An infusion of 1 g/kg of dextrose plus 0.25 units/kg soluble insulin is frequently used to improve myocardial function and to decrease hyperkalaemia. Frequent blood sugar estimations must be made when using this regimen.

Post-resuscitation care

Following resuscitation the child must be carefully transferred to a paediatric critical care facility. Ventilation and inotropic support may need to be continued, and a urinary catheter should be inserted to estimate urine output. Arterial blood-gas, plasma electrolyte measurements, and a chest X-ray should be repeated, and any abnormal findings should be corrected.

Careful monitoring of the child's temperature must be commenced. Hypothermia will cause additional strain on the cardiovascular system. Hypothermia is poorly tolerated in the baby and the small infant, and it is therefore vitally important to maintain the body temperature of the child during resuscitation. A warming mattress, an overhead infrared heater, heating inspired gases, and warming intravenous fluids will all help to correct and maintain body temperature.

Drug and fluid administration

During paediatric resuscitation all drugs and fluids are given in a dose calculated per kilogram body weight. Unfortunately, in the acute resuscitation event there is never time to weigh the child, and estimations of the weight can be notoriously inaccurate. If the age of the child is known then a more accurate estimation of the weight can be made using the following data:

- Infants double their birth weight in 5 months.
- Infants treble their birth weight in 1 year.
- Between 1 and 9 years, weight (kg) = (age + 4) × 2.
- Between 7 and 12, weight (kg) = age × 3.

Probably the simplest method of estimating weight, drug dosages, and tracheal tube size and length is to use Fig. 9.8. Here, a simple measurement of the child's length gives information on the tracheal tube size and length (y-axis) and drug doses (x-axis). The importance of this diagram cannot be overemphasized. Simple mistakes in calculating dosages or the conversion of drug doses to millilitres of solution to be administered can have fatal consequences.

Further reading

1. American Heart Association (1986). Standards and Guidelines for Cardiopulmonary Resuscitation (CPR and Emergency Cardiac Care (ECC). *Journal of the American Medical Association*, **255**, 2954–69.
2. Ludwig, S. and Kettrick, R. G. (1983). Paediatric resuscitation for the non-paediatrician. In *Clinics in emergency medicine: Resuscitation* Vol. 2, pp. 101–12. Churchill Livingstone, Edinburgh.
3. Oakley, P. (1988). Inaccuracy and delay in decision making in paediatric resuscitation, and a proposed chart to reduce error, *British Medical Journal*, **297**, 817–19.
4. Orlowski, J. P. (1986). Optimum position of external cardiac compression in infants and young children. *Annals of Emergency Medicine*, **15**, 667–73.
5. Phillips, G. W. L. and Zideman, D. A. (1986). Relation of infant heart to the sternum: its significance in cardiopulmonary resuscitation. *Lancet*, **i**, 1024–5.
6. Seidel, J. (1986). A needs assessment of advanced life support and emergency medical services in the paediatric patient: state of the art. *Circulation*, **74** (Suppl. IV), 129–33.
7. Zaritsky, A. (1986). Advanced paediatric life support: state of the art. *Circulation*, **74** (Suppl. IV), 124–8.
8. Zideman, D. A. (1990). Resuscitation of infants and children. In *ABC of resuscitation*, 2nd edn, (ed. T. R. Evans), pp. 43–7. British Medical Journal, London.

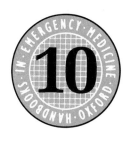

CHAPTER 10

Who to resuscitate and post-resuscitation care

Key points in who to resuscitate and post-resuscitation care

1 Decisions regarding whether or not to resuscitate in-patients should be made in advance.

2 The decision to cease a resuscitation attempt should be agreed between the team members.

3 The most senior member of the cardiac arrest team should discuss the outcome with the relatives.

4 Relatives may wish to discuss the events surrounding an unsuccessful resuscitation weeks or months after the event—medical staff should make themselves available for this.

5 Post-resuscitation care should take place in consultation with the intensive care team.

The decision to resuscitate

In-patients

The decision to resuscitate or not can be difficult. To avoid confusion, if a cardiac arrest should occur in an in-patient, a decision as to whether resuscitation is appropriate should have been made in advance. A variety of factors will influence this decision, but it should be reached by consensus with the medical team involved, together with their nursing colleagues, the patient's relatives, and, if appropriate, the patient himself or herself. The patient's illness, age, and general quality of life will influence the decision, and various guidelines have been suggested, namely: resuscitation may be withheld for a patient whose general health has been declining progressively over many years, or, for instance, when even if the patient were resuscitated, the quality of life would be so poor as to be regarded by most as unacceptable. Decisions made for in-patients should be understood clearly by nursing and medical staff, and recorded in both the medical and nursing case notes.

In the Accident and Emergency Department

For patients brought to the Accident and Emergency Department in cardiac arrest, resuscitation should be started, or continued, until the history becomes clear.

Box 10.1 ● For patients brought into A&E

'Resuscitate first, ask questions during and after.'

It may be that a considerable period of cardiopulmonary standstill occurred before resuscitation was commenced in the field in an elderly patient whose previous quality of life was, in any event, poor. This will preclude a prolonged attempt. Such decisions are difficult, and must be made in a sensitive fashion during the resuscitation attempt. They should involve all members of the cardiac arrest team, including the nursing staff. It is possible under these circumstances that a disagreement may occur amongst team members. If this is the case then the Team Leader should agree to continue the attempt, but with a very definite end-point. This end-point should be agreed. For instance: 'We will give one more bolus of adrenaline, and if this asystolic patient does not begin to fibrillate after three minutes of massage and ventilation then we will abandon the resuscitation attempt.' This will, it is hoped, satisfy the team, with all members feeling that everything possible was done in attempting to resuscitate the patient.

In general, therefore, a decision **not** to resuscitate should only be taken when all the details of the patient's history are clear and have been discussed amongst all concerned, and the decision has been reached in harmony. In other circumstances, particularly in the A&E Department, resuscitation should be commenced and continued until details become clear.

Post-resuscitation care following unsuccessful resuscitation

Informing the relatives

If the patient does not survive it is the Team Leader's responsibility, as the most senior doctor present, to inform the relatives immediately. All too often this task is left to the most junior doctor. This is to be condemned.

When talking to the relatives the Team Leader should be accompanied by a qualified member of the nursing staff. He or she should be in possession of the patient's notes, and should clearly identify each relative's name and their relationship to the patient. The conversation should be conducted in a room designated as a Relatives Room in the A&E Department or, on a ward, ideally in the Sister's office.

Having identified the relative the doctor should inform him or her that the patient, who should be referred to by name, **has died**. It is of paramount importance that relatives are left in no doubt as to the final outcome, because powerful forces of denial may be aroused in them. These denial forces should be

> **Box 10.2** ● Check-list after unsuccessful resuscitation attempt
>
> - Relatives
> - General practitioner
> - Coroner/Procurator Fiscal
> - Valuables
> - Religious needs
> - Cardiac arrest team debriefing

aborted at the earliest opportunity by plain speaking. Phrases such as 'passed away' or 'gone to a better place' might be interpreted by the relatives as meaning that the patient has been transferred to another hospital. There must be no room for such confusion.

It may be appropriate at this stage to ask the relatives if they wish to see a member of a religious fraternity. Pastors of most faiths are usually readily available on call. The relatives may also wish to see the patient. This should be encouraged and arranged, either in the resuscitation room or, preferably, in the Chapel of Rest adjacent to the hospital mortuary. Naturally there are official duties that the relatives will have to perform in these circumstances; but these may often, with the Coroner's consent, be left until the following day, after the initial shock has subsided.

The death of a child is a special circumstance, and a paediatrician should always be present when the relatives are informed.

Having concluded the discussion with the relatives, the doctor should state that he or she is always available, months or even years later, to talk about the case again. A standard form, with the names of the relevant medical and nursing staff, together with a means of contact—ideally direct-dial hospital telephone numbers—is helpful. Not infrequently, the relatives will have questions, which seemed inappropriate at the time, that they may wish to ask later. These subsequent discussions often prove tremendously helpful for the relatives, and the doctor should make herself or himself readily available if contacted.

Box 10.3 ● Requirements for the Relatives Room

- Quiet
- Comfortable chairs
- Telephone with an outside line
- Tea and coffee

Cardiac arrest team debriefing

Following the initial discussion with the relatives the Team Leader should make time, with the rest of the cardiac arrest team, for a debrief session. Aspects of the patient's management during the arrest can be discussed, problems that arose can be solved, and subsequent resuscitation attempts can be further improved.

Finally, the patient's general practitioner must be informed. He will appreciate knowing not only about the death, but also what the relatives have been told.

Post-resuscitation care following a successful resuscitation attempt

Stabilize ventilation

If the patient survives a cardiac arrest on a ward or in the A&E Department, arrangements must be made for his or her continuing care, usually on the Cardiac or Intensive Care Unit. Basic support requirements should be checked and ventilation should be stabilized. The anaesthetist will usually be entirely responsible for this part of the patient's management, as well as for assessing the patient's oxygenation and acid–base balance, using blood-gas measurements and pulse oximetry.

Monitoring the patient

The patient's cardiac rhythm and haemodynamic status must be monitored, with an ECG monitor and by the use of a central venous pressure line. If circumstances permit, also use an arterial pressure line with a wave-form read out. Urgent venous blood specimens should be sent for measurements of serum potassium, glucose levels, and full blood count.

Problems of transfer

The details of transfer should be organized, and accompanying doctors and nursing staff should be designated so that the patient receives continuing intensive care during the journey to CCU or ICU. Transfer within a hospital is hazardous, and the most senior doctor should, therefore, be present. The patient must be transferred with a portable monitor/defibrillator and airway, ventilation, and suction equipment, as well as all necessary drugs. Notes should be prepared and the receiving team should be alerted to the patient's history, particularly his or her recent resuscitation history.

Communicating with relatives

The relatives must not be forgotten; the Team Leader must inform them of the successful initial outcome of resuscitation, while at the same time warning them that the patient's health can, at best be described as critical. Arrangements should be made with nursing staff for the relatives to be taken to the CCU or ICU some little time after the patient has arrived. They should then be introduced to the unit's staff at the earliest opportunity.

Early intensive care in A&E

While a bed is being prepared on the ICU it is useful, in consultation with the Intensive Care consultant, to initiate some aspects of intensive care in the Resuscitation Room of the Accident Department. Particular attention must be paid to $P\text{CO}_2$, blood glucose, control of convulsions, and the use of thrombolysis.

Blood gas control

The $P\text{CO}_2$ should ideally be kept low, in the range of 3.8–4.2 $k\text{P}_a$. This can be achieved by hyperventilating the patient, but blood gases should be carefully monitored, because if the $P\text{CO}_2$ becomes lower than 3.8 $k\text{P}_a$ paradoxical cerebral vasoconstriction may result.

208 • Who to resuscitate and post-resuscitation care

Serum glucose control

Blood glucose levels should be maintained at a normal level. A high blood glucose supply to the ischaemic post-arrest brain will encourage anaerobic metabolism and the production of a lactic acidosis. This may lead to further brain damage. A normal blood glucose level will, however, be needed for normal metabolism.

Control of convulsions

Epileptiform convulsions may occur and must be controlled. Intravenous benzodiazepines should be administered. Diazepines given intravenously at a rate of 2.5 mg every 30 seconds and up to 20 mg in an adult will usually control convulsions but may cause respiratory depression and hypotension. When the fits have been controlled, blood gas levels should be estimated. Prophylactically, phenytoin in a dose of 10–15 mg/kg may be given intravenously over one hour, as a loading dose, which will need to be followed on the ICU by a dosage of 300 mg of phenytoin daily.

Considering thrombolysis

If the patient, on presentation to the A&E Department, had suffered a myocardial infarction precipitating cardiac arrest, then thrombolysis should be considered, providing there are no exclusion factors. It is generally accepted that thrombolysis will be excluded if vigorous resuscitation has taken place, particularly with prolonged, energetic external cardiac compression (see p. 81).

It must be stressed that these measures are more appropriate in the setting of the ICU; but in some circumstances a bed may not be immediately available.

Cardiac arrest team debriefing

In the same way as for an unsuccessful resuscitation attempt, a debrief should still occur following a successful resuscitation, as there is always room for improvement in the management of patients suffering cardiac arrest.

In practice, there will frequently not be time in busy hospital practice for a full team debriefing. The Resuscitation Training Officer (RTO) can be invaluable in auditing resuscitation attempts and assisting in the debriefing and education of the resuscitation team. A standard form is useful in collecting data from resuscitation attempt records. This should detail which medical and nursing staff were present, the patient's history and the cause of arrest, and details of drugs, defibrillating shocks, and methods of airway care used during the attempt. Outcome and, if the patient survived, details of the consultant and ward where post-resuscitation care is to be continued should be recorded. In unsuccessful attempts the coroner's post-mortem report should be collected at a later date. Hospital-wide policy changes felt necessary as a result of such continuous audit can be effected via the Resuscitation Committee.

Further reading

1. Cathcart, F. (1988). Seeing the body after death. *British Medical Journal*, **297**, 997.
2. Holmberg, S. and Ekström, L. (1992). Ethics and practicalities of resuscitation—a statement for the ERC. *Resuscitation*, **24**, 239–44.
3. Kentsch, M. *et al.* (1990). Early prediction of prognosis in out-of-hospital cardiac arrest. *Intensive Care Medicine*, **6**, 378–83.
4. Lo, B. and Jonsen, A. R. (1980). Clinical decisions to limit treatment. *Annals of Internal Medicine*, **93**, 764–8.
5. Mullie, A., Buylaert, W., Michom, N., Verbruggen, H., Corne, L., De Cock, R., *et al.* Predictive value of Glasgow Coma Score for awakening after out-of-hospital cardiac arrest. *Lancet*, **i**, 137–40.
6. McLauchlan, C. A. J. (1990). Handling distressed relatives and breaking bad news. In *ABC of major trauma*, (ed. D. Skinner, P. Driscoll, and R. Earlam), pp. 102–6; *British Medical Journal*, **301**, 1145–9.
7. Weston, C. F. M., Penny, W. J. and Julian, D. G. (1994). Guidelines for the early management of patients with myocardial infarction. *British Medical Journal*, **308**, 767–71.

Index

ADVANCED CARDIAC LIFE SUPPORT

Responsive? → No → **Breathing?** → No → **Pulse?** → No → **Start CPR** 2:15

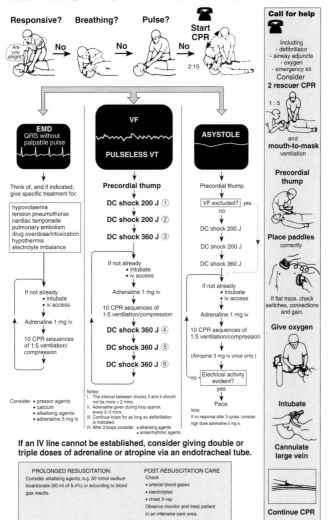

Call for help

Including
- defibrillator
- airway adjuncts
- oxygen
- emergency kit

Consider **2 rescuer CPR**

1:5

and **mouth-to-mask** ventilation

Precordial thump

Place paddles correctly

If flat trace, check switches, connections and gain.

Give oxygen

Intubate

Cannulate large vein

Continue CPR

© Copyright ERC 1992

EMD
QRS without palpable pulse

Think of, and if indicated, give specific treatment for:

hypovolaemia
tension pneumothorax
cardiac tamponade
pulmonary embolism
drug overdose/intoxication
hypothermia
electrolyte imbalance

If not already
- intubate
- iv access

Adrenaline 1 mg iv

10 CPR sequences of 1:5 ventilation/compression

Consider
- pressor agents
- calcium
- alkalising agents
- adrenaline 5 mg iv

VF
PULSELESS VT

Precordial thump

DC shock 200 J ①

DC shock 200 J ②

DC shock 360 J ③

If not already
- intubate
- iv access

Adrenaline 1 mg iv

10 CPR sequences of 1:5 ventilation/compression

DC shock 360 J ④

DC shock 360 J ⑤

DC shock 360 J ⑥

Notes:
I. The interval between shocks 3 and 4 should not be more > 2 mins.
II. Adrenaline given during loop approx. every 2–3 mins.
III. Continue loops for as long as defibrillation is indicated.
IV. After 3 loops consider • alkalising agents • antiarrhythmic agents

---

ASYSTOLE

Precordial thump

VF excluded? yes

no

DC shock 200 J

DC shock 200 J

DC shock 360 J

If not already
- intubate
- iv access

Adrenaline 1 mg iv

10 CPR sequences of 1:5 ventilation/compression

(Atropine 3 mg iv *once only*)

no — Electrical activity evident?

yes

Pace

Note:
If no response after 3 cycles, consider high dose adrenaline 5 mg iv.

If an IV line cannot be established, consider giving double or triple doses of adrenaline or atropine via an endotracheal tube.

PROLONGED RESUSCITATION:
Consider alkalising agents, e.g. 50 mmol sodium bicarbonate (50 ml of 8.4%) or according to blood gas results.

POST RESUSCITATION CARE
Check
- arterial blood gases
- electrolytes
- chest X-ray
Observe monitor and treat patient in an intensive care area.

European Resuscitation Council
in co-operation with
Resuscitation Council (UK)